CW01614389

Advanced Removable Partial Dentures

Advanced Removable Partial Dentures

James S. Brudvik, DDS, FACP
Professor Emeritus of Prosthodontics
University of Washington
School of Dentistry
Seattle, Washington

quintessence books

Quintessence Publishing Co, Inc
Chicago, Berlin, London, Tokyo, Paris, Barcelona, São Paulo,
Moscow, Prague, and Warsaw

Library of Congress Cataloging-in-Publication Data

Brudvik, James S.
Advanced removable partial dentures / James S. Brudvik.
p. cm.
Includes index.
ISBN 0-86715-351-2 (hard cover)
1. Partial dentures, Removable. I. Title.
[DNLM: 1. Denture, Partial, Removable. WU 515 B888a 1999]
RK665.B78 1999
617.6'92—dc21
DNLM/DLC
for Library of Congress

99-21231
CIP

quintessence books

© 1999 Quintessence Publishing Co, Inc

Quintessence Publishing Co, Inc
551 Kimberly Drive
Carol Stream, Illinois 60188

All rights reserved. This book or any part thereof may not be reproduced, stored in a retrieval system, or transmitted in any form or by any means, electronic, mechanical, photocopying, or otherwise, without prior written permission of the publisher.

Editor: Lori Bateman
Design/Production: Michael Shanahan

Printed in the USA

Contents

Preface

The removable partial denture has always been my special challenge in dentistry. As a clinician, researcher, dental laboratory director, lecturer, and mentor, I have spent almost 35 years trying to come to grips with the complexities of this form of prosthodontic treatment. I would estimate that 20% of partial wearers are more than just a little dissatisfied with their denture. Unlike with the fixed partial denture, the patient has the option of removing the prosthesis at the slightest hint of discomfort, physical or mental. Given the actual state of practice—the dentist does only the occasional partial denture with almost total reliance on the dental laboratory for design as well as construction—I am most pessimistic as to the effect of this, or any other text on the subject.

While there are a number of excellent basic texts on the removable partial denture, they are all directed toward the undergraduate dental student. I have not found anything that I can use as an advanced text for the graduate student and study club participant who wishes to pursue this form of therapy at the highest level. After years of being asked if I had ever considered putting my lecture material in written form and protesting that I did not have the time, my partial retirement from the University of Washington School of Dentistry has made my excuses no longer valid.

This work is not intended to be a textbook in the classical sense. It is, rather, a monograph on the removable partial denture, written with the expectation that the reader will already have covered the basics of the partial denture and is now ready to take a more sophisticated look at this treatment modality. It does not have a bibliography, and the illustrations consist of drawings that I have placed on countless blackboards over the years in an attempt to make things clear to my students. What follows are my thoughts as they have evolved over these years of practice and teaching in this fascinating area.

While I take complete responsibility for the content of this work, I have been aided in the writing by my friend and coworker,

Janine Nemerever Coates, who, as program coordinator of the Graduate Program in Prosthodontics, has long stood watch over my faulty grammar and sentence structure. I have also had the help of Dr Alex Shor, presently in our graduate program, who has reviewed the entire book to provide insight and guidance from the eyes of the potential readership.

This book is dedicated to my graduate students—past, present, and hopefully future—who provide, on a daily basis, the joy of seeing someone learn. It is also dedicated to my longtime friend and colleague, the eminent functional anatomist, Professor Jean Romerowski of the University of Paris, VII, who has been an inspiration in this matter as in so many other endeavors over the years.

Introduction

The removable partial denture has long been considered an inferior means of replacing missing teeth and associated structures when compared to the fixed partial denture. Some have even spoken of it as a stepping stone to a complete denture. The old rhyme, "Little RPD, don't you cry. You'll be a CD by and by" may best express our feelings toward this treatment modality. Many surveys published over the years in our journals indicate that dentistry does a rather poor job with the RPD. These reports testify to the fact that most RPDs are created entirely by the technician with a minimum of input from the clinician in the form of mouth preparation or design.

Dental schools make a serious effort to teach the subject, and excellent texts for the undergraduate are available. Nonetheless, the state of removable partial dentures seen in the commercial laboratories and in the cross-sectional studies available to us indicates that, in general, partials are poorly designed and constructed and poorly maintained.

Therefore, it is no wonder that patients dislike their partials to the point of not wearing them and, if they can afford alternative treatment, request it routinely. It has been my experience that the patient who states, "I had a partial once and couldn't wear it!" most likely had a substandard prosthesis; when treated with a state-of-the-art partial denture, the patient would likely find it tolerable and easily accept the limitations of this form of tooth and tissue replacement.

Plainly stated, there is a dramatic difference between the standard RPD and the one that approaches the state of the art as we know it today. It is in the attempt to create that quality removable partial denture that this book is written. It is intended to serve as a guide to both graduate students in prosthodontics and concerned general practitioners—to challenge them to think of the removable appliance as they would the fixed partial denture, with all the same considerations of soft tissue management, caries control, periodontal support, orthodontic therapy, and implant involvement. In almost every clinical situation, the patient who requires a removable partial denture will have a need for some form of fixed prosthodontics as well, from a simple bonded rest to the most complex precision attachments extending from fixed units.

Philosophy of Care

What makes a successful RPD? At the risk of oversimplification, one could say that the successful removable appliance need be only four things:

1. *Strong*, in that it does not wear, break, distort, or come apart when worn.
2. *Retentive*, so that it remains in position in the patient's mouth during use and gives the patient confidence that it will continue to do so over the life of the partial.
3. *Esthetic*, to satisfy the patient's expectations without undue evidence of its presence.
4. *Pain-free*, meaning that it does not cause discomfort when in the mouth for the short term and that it causes no long-term damage to either hard or soft tissue over the life of the partial.

If these four requirements can be met, the partial stands a good chance of long-term success. Unfortunately, the success of the partial in and of itself does not guarantee the long-term health of the remaining teeth and soft tissues. Maintenance, therefore, becomes the primary factor in the long-term success of the treatment. The profession has usually substituted concern over the type of clasp to be used for the more fundamental requirements of regularly scheduled recall and appropriate maintenance. Preparing the mouth to its very best state of health before starting prosthodontic procedures and then keeping the tissues in that state of health over the life of the partial is far more important than any design considerations. It has become obvious to me that a partial denture in a healthy mouth, assuming that it meets our four requirements, will be successful regardless of its design. Rest placement and clasp design, interesting as they may be to argue over from a theoretical point of view, are simply not germane to the real question of what makes a successful removable partial denture. Suppositions derived from bench studies do not necessarily transfer to the clinical realities of long-term care.

How long should a properly designed, constructed, and maintained RPD last? Good evidence exists that this state-of-the-art partial could be expected to last a minimum of 10 years, assuming that the patient was seen at regular intervals and that both the mouth and the partial received the indicated maintenance. Partials providing good service for 20 years are not unheard of, although the long-term maintenance requirements increase dramatically after 10 years.

The construction of the removable partial denture, more than any other form of dental therapy, is almost always delegated to the dental laboratory since the equipment required to produce an acceptable cast framework is not going to be found in the dental office. In many cases, the clinician may have never even met the technicians creating the prostheses. This fact requires that the clinicians maintain control by inserting themselves into the process at the critical steps in construction. These steps will be covered in depth in this book.

Since the actual construction is delegated, the average clinician is apt to have very little confidence or experience in these matters and is likely to take the technician's view of the design and construction process, a view that will be more mechanical than biological. The wise clinician will make a point of remaining in close contact with the technician and bringing these auxiliaries into the clinical aspects of care whenever possible.

The modern removable partial denture combines fixed and removable prosthodontics and requires a thorough understanding of both aspects of care by the clinician and by the technician. Unfortunately, the evolution of the dental laboratory industry has separated technicians into often isolated specialties: complete dentures, removable partial dentures, and fixed partial dentures. The technician who is knowledgeable in all areas is a vanishing breed. To direct the construction of the most sophisticated restorations, the clinician must assume the responsibility of coordinating the laboratory phases. This text is intended to set standards of care for the comprehensive management of the partially edentulous patient who will require some form of a removable restoration.

1

Patient Evaluation, Diagnosis, and Treatment Planning

The obvious first step in treatment for the partially edentulous patient includes the gathering of diagnostic data and those diagnostic procedures commonly grouped under the heading of treatment planning. These procedures must also address the prognosis, with and without treatment, of individual teeth as well as the mouth as a whole. An integral part of the required diagnostic data will be the information gathered from a diagnostic wax-up and set-up that includes a tentative RPD design as well. It may well be that the diagnostic phase is second only to maintenance as an indicator of long-term success.

Initial Examination

The following sequence represents the basic information that must be obtained before treatment planning can occur:

1. Identification of the patient's chief complaint
2. Head and neck examination
3. TMJ evaluation to include sounds and mouth opening
4. Intraoral examination of both soft and hard tissues with emphasis on cancer screening
5. Accurate and complete charting of:
   - *Caries*
   - *Existing restorations*
   - *Periodontal tissues, to include pocket probing, and mobility, and general bone levels*
   - *Pulp vitality, especially of potential abutment teeth*
   - *Radiographic findings of periapical films and a pantograph (in cases where jaw discrepancies and malocclusions are obvious, a lateral head film with tracing and evaluation can be requested with orthodontic consultation)*
   - *Occlusal contacts, centric and eccentric*

6. Additional procedures sometimes indicated:
   - *Diet analysis*
   - *Caries risk assessment*
7. Impressions for diagnostic casts
8. Interocclusal jaw relation record (if indicated)
9. Shade and mold selection

The need for this diagnostic data should be obvious to any clinician. Unfortunately, the planning for the average RPD seldom includes all these issues and, as a result, the treatment is compromised from the very beginning. There is no point even considering the "design" portion of the treatment plan until this information is available and has received some consideration and reflection.

Decision Making for RPD Treatment Planning

A series of questions (in no particular order) must be addressed as part of the evaluation of the gathered data.

Is a removable partial denture indicated/necessary for this patient at this time?

Would the patient be better served with a fixed or an implant-retained prosthesis, and can the increase in cost of care be justified?

What prosthodontic/restorative needs are apparent in the opposing arch, and how will their treatment affect the removable partial denture?

Are the hard and soft tissues that would relate to a removable appliance acceptable (in an ideal state of health) at this time, or will they require preprosthetic therapy? This could include everything from orthognathic surgery to a bonded metal rest. Will the abutment teeth provide all the required support, or will additional support be required from the soft tissues of the edentulous areas (stress relief)?

Are the patient's expectations achievable?

Will the patient be able to provide the required level of home care that will be necessary for long-term success?

Should ideal treatment be modified because of age, chronic systemic disease, or psychological factors?

Most, if not all, of these questions should be addressed as a part of the initial examination. Some will require direct questioning of the patient. Others may only need to be a part of the clinician's thought process but should be considered while the patient is still present. Some questions will result in referrals to other specialists and/or additional diagnostic tests.

The wise clinician will not give the patient any definitive plan or fee at the time of the initial examination. It is far better to tell the patient that no intelligent response can be made until all of the diagnostic data have been evaluated and any required consultations obtained.

Preliminary Impressions

The quality of the initial impressions and the casts that result from them, although diagnostic only, need to be of far higher quality than that normally seen. Most every specialist in removable prosthodontics has, while attending a meeting or seminar, been approached for help in treatment planning a case. A plaster cast is pulled from a pocket, usually without a decent base, full of blebs and voids and with no evidence of ever having been on a dental surveyor. "I apologize for this cast, but can you help me with a design?"

The preliminary impression and resultant cast should be of the same quality as the final impression as far as extensions, hard and soft tissue details, and integrity of the occlusal surface are concerned. This impression should be considered as a trial impression for the final. Tray size is evaluated, patient compliance with instructions noted, ease of placement discovered, and the patient's ability to sit still during the set of the alginate evaluated. Everything that can be learned from this impression will aid the clinician in making an accurate final impression.

Sometimes no stock tray will adequately fit the mouth, indicating that a custom tray will have to be included in preparation for the final impression. Modification of the stock tray with wax or compound may be necessary to allow the impression of border tissues or high palatal vault. All these issues must be evaluated when the preliminary impression is made so that the clinician can concentrate on accuracy of the hard tissues in the final impression.

Alginate can be expected to give overextended borders due to its consistency when properly mixed. Under no circumstances should the powder-water ratio be changed to reduce the viscosity of the mix. Rather, the amount of alginate required to make a quality impression should be carefully estimated and only that amount placed in the tray. Alginate must be placed into the critical areas: rest seats, guiding planes, soft tissue undercuts, etc. One cannot count on the material flowing to these areas of its own accord. The material can be placed with the finger or injected using a syringe, but in no instance should the tray be placed in the mouth until all critical areas are wiped with alginate. Borders should be filled using a syringe. A plastic 35 cc Monojet syringe with 10 to 15 cc of alginate will work well in most situations. The critical areas are buccal to the tuberosities and the retromylohyoid space, places where voids are often found in the completed impression. Another advantage of placing alginate in the mouth before seating the tray is that less material (the total mix minus the 10 to 15 cc) need be placed in the tray, resulting in increased visibility for tray placement.

Whenever possible, the stock tray is modified by adding wax or compound to allow a minimum of 0.25 inch of alginate around all critical structures. A common problem with alginate is overseating of the tray, resulting in less than the required 0.25 inch of material over the occlusal surfaces. Stops can be placed in the tray using hard wax or dental compound to restrict the overseating. Unfortunately, the area of the stop will often be distorted due to the minimal alginate present. The required occlusal spacing may be obtained by placing the empty tray in the mouth, seating it to contact with the occlusal surfaces, and evaluating the relative position of the handle to the lips when the tray is lifted the 0.25 inch. In making the impression, the tray is seated to that lifted position and held in place until the impression is set.

When the impression is removed from the mouth, it must be rinsed and lightly dried, then inspected for tears and any evidence of the material breaking free from the rimlock or retentive holes. When using a rimlock tray, excess alginate should be cut from the borders with a sharp knife so that the edge of the tray can be seen and the retention of the alginate verified.

Alginate is clearly an abused impression material, but it is the material of choice for both preliminary and final impressions for the removable partial denture. Seldom is the alginate mixed for the manufacturer's recommended time. Likewise, it is often not allowed time for a complete set before removal from the mouth. Many inaccurate impressions can be traced to the patient's inability to remain motionless during the setting phase. When the time in the mouth has been altered by using very cold water or not mixing for the usual 60 seconds, the patient is forced to remain motionless for longer than necessary. Since alginate does not set all at once but in scattered islands, any movement by clinician or patient during the setting period runs the risk of reorienting the partially set material and producing a distorted impression. Ideally, the set should begin promptly after the tray is in its proper position and any border molding has occurred. Alginate mixed with the proper measure of room-temperature (65°F to 70°F) water will allow roughly a minute for loading the tray and placing it in the mouth before the set begins. Optimal gelation time should be between 3 and 4 minutes using 68°F water. The patient is instructed to remain motionless during this time. The initial impression gives the clinician the opportunity to test the patient's ability in this regard to increase the probability that the final impression will be accurate. Should the patient move during the final impression, it must be remade and the patient informed again of his or her part in this procedure.

If the mixing of the alginate is incomplete, a reduction of up to 50% in the strength of the gel can be expected. On the other hand, alginate mixed beyond the manufacturer's stated time will have a reduced gel strength since the forming gels will be broken. Mechanical mixing devices, including vacuum mixing, are more apt to provide consistency and thereby accuracy, and should be considered as essential instrumentation. Hand mixing for the full minute required by most manufacturers is not that easily accomplished and, as a result, the mixing time is seldom fully utilized.

Alginate adhesives must be considered essential for all final impressions, but since they are not easy to remove from the tray, they are not required for the diagnostic impression. When a stock rimlock tray is used, however, care must be taken to force the alginate into the rimlock with the spatula when loading the tray. Once this has been done, the alginate is not likely to pop free of the lock. Nevertheless, the impression should be carefully inspected before pouring so that if a separation has occurred, the set alginate can be replaced in the lock of the tray. While this maneuver would be unacceptable for a final impression, it will normally produce a cast that is accurate enough for diagnostic procedures.

Once the impression has been removed from the mouth, the following series of steps, performed in this order, will maximize chances for an accurate diagnostic cast:

1. Rinse the impression under running water.
2. Using a cotton tip, gently clean the tooth impressions. (Plaque and other oral debris, if left in the impression, will reduce the surface hardness of the resultant cast, since the surface hardening agents in the alginate must come into contact

with the dental stone for maximum hardness to be achieved.)

3. Blow excess fluid from the impression and evaluate the impression under good light for tears and defects.
4. With an indelible pencil or other marker, trace the outline of the proposed denture on the alginate. Since the patient is still in the chair, extensions can be quickly verified. Should contours seen in the mouth and essential to the construction not be present in the impression, the decision to remake the impression will not require an additional appointment. Attempts to identify denture base extensions from a stone cast days after the impression was made often lead to problems with extensions and will never be as accurate as those determined via this method of drawing on the alginate impression.
5. The technique used to pour the preliminary impression is immaterial. Any approach that results in a dense cast with no voids and a base suitable for mounting in the dental surveyor will suffice for diagnostic purposes. As a minimum, the cast should be neatly trimmed and all blebs removed, since this cast may well be seen by the patient as well as by the technician. A neat diagnostic cast with a careful design, properly drawn, goes a long way toward indicating that the clinician really does know the standards. My experience has been that technicians are impressed when they see a quality diagnostic cast.

Preprosthetic Therapy

Determining the level of mouth preparation required is an essential element of the state-of-the-art removable partial denture. Mouth preparation is usually interpreted to mean the creation of rest preparations on some of the remaining teeth. Unfortunately, reviews of cases submitted to the dental laboratories show that many mouths have not even this level of mouth preparation.

For the modern RPD, mouth preparation will cover any therapy required to bring the mouth to optimum health and to modify tissue in such a manner as to make the final prosthesis ideal. Obviously, a removable appliance can be made to accept the mouth as it presents. In fact, most of the RPDs seen in any review of prosthetic treatment will fall into this category, with occlusal plane discrepancies, malocclusions, little or no recontouring of teeth, and the like. A discussion of the basic therapies for mouth preparation at this point in the treatment planning process is necessary to fully develop the concept of ideal mouth preparation.

While the sequencing of the actual care is a critical issue, the sequencing of consultations is not. The prosthodontist will almost always manage the restorative dental examination and caries risk assessment. Nutritional evaluation for those patients with obvious active caries may be referred to a nutritionist, although there are computer software programs available so that a diet survey, completed over a 5-day period by the patient, can be analyzed without special training in most cases (eg, Food Processor Plus 6.0 ESHA Research, Salem, Oregon).

The periodontal examination is a different matter, since most prosthodontists have a network of periodontists with whom they exchange referrals. No matter how the data are gathered, a baseline of pocket depths, furcation involvement, plaque scores, mobility levels, and general periodontal soft tissue conditions must be made. Baseline data of this magnitude provide the clinician with a starting point for referrals as well as protection for medicolegal matters.

Endodontic referrals are apt to be more common, especially those regarding existing endodontic restorations. Re-treatment decisions can greatly affect the treatment plan, both in regard to abutment selection and to total cost of care.

Orthodontic and oral and maxillofacial surgical consultations are almost always case specific and may not always be necessary, although to plan treatment without them the clinician must be assured that they will not contribute to the care of the patient. A large number of cases will require minor tooth movement to align the arch and to establish the ideal occlusal plane. Often these consultations can best be done after a preliminary treatment plan and design have been established.

Along with the periodontal examination, the evaluation of existing restorations and tooth contours is critical to our treatment. In far too many instances, restorations of marginal quality are left in the mouth and the partial built around them.

Once the above information has been gathered, the clinical findings can be summarized as a part of the patient's record and included in the treatment plan letter. A diagnosis and prognosis of the mouth with and without treatment can also be established. At this point, the diagnostic casts, radiographs, and periodontal charting are reviewed together, and the cast is "surveyed" to determine the RPD options. The treatment plan and the patient's informed consent letter can only be completed after the tentative design of the final appliance has been established.

Is all this really necessary? Must a written treatment plan and consent letter be given to the patient? Should we make an orthodontic consult a part of our chain of diagnostic procedures? The answer to these and similar questions is, of course, most certainly *yes*! The type of treatment described in this book—the partial denture at the most advanced level—does require more work, both in planning and execution. The results are, very obviously, worth our time and our best efforts.

2

Removable Partial Denture Design

Ever since the publication of Dr W. Frantz's study of the variations in partial denture design (J Prosthet Dent, 1973), I have been troubled by the seemingly total lack of consensus on the design of a conventional partial denture. I can understand that there would be some different approaches to any partial design, but to find that there is apparently no commonly held approach that would result in a minimum of variations is troubling. It may well be that the average clinician simply does not have sufficient repetitions of similar partially edentulous situations to develop a consistent philosophy for designing a partial denture.

For any situation where there are inadequate repetitions or where the consequences of overlooking a particular step are unacceptable, the development of a checklist, not unlike that used by the pilot of an airplane, is in order. The checklist that I have used and taught for many years is based on what I believe to be the most logical approach to determining the design of any removable partial situation. It focuses on clinical rather than laboratory decision making and is broken down into the following categories, always in this order, since it ranks the components, or elements of design, by clinical importance.

RPD Design Checklist

1. Abutments and rests
2. Connectors, major and minor
3. Resin retention
4. Retention, clasp or attachment

Elements of Design

Abutments and Rests

The relationship between the abutment tooth and the framework is the most important of all design and construction considerations. In keeping with this thought, the selection of the remaining teeth to be used as abutments becomes critical. An abutment is defined as any tooth that bears

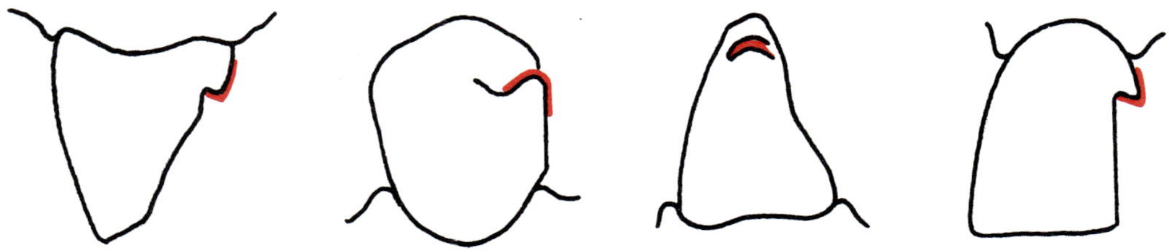

Fig 2-1 Positive rest forms (< 90 degrees).

the vertical and oblique loads placed upon the partial through positive rests. Positive rests are defined as rests that form acute angles with the minor connectors that connect them to the major connector. With a rest/connector angle of less than 90 degrees, the partial cannot get away from the tooth and the tooth cannot move away from the partial (Fig 2-1).

Whenever possible, missing anterior teeth are to be replaced with fixed partial dentures, leaving the RPD to replace posterior teeth. Attempting to replace both anterior and posterior teeth on the same casting is a compromise that may affect both esthetics and abutment stability. As an additional benefit of anterior fixed replacements, the abutment castings will be given ideal contours to support the posterior partial and to allow the elimination of buccal clasp arms. A variety of precision and semiprecision attachments can be incorporated in these abutment crowns to eliminate anterior clasping.

Selection of the abutment teeth begins with an evaluation of the strength of each tooth. As a general rule, we must consider the strongest remaining teeth first and then progress to weaker teeth as we decide upon the number of teeth necessary to support the partial. Whether or not a tooth is ultimately selected to be clasped as well as rested is immaterial at this time. It is always preferable to include more abutments rather than fewer, since the only negative aspect of extra abutments is that they make the casting more complex in geometry and thus decrease the likelihood of a perfect fit. Obviously, the number of teeth to be replaced is related to the number of abutments needed for support.

The type of rest preparation to be placed upon the selected abutment tooth is generally obvious: occlusal rests for posterior teeth and cingulum rests for incisors. Since there is often inadequate enamel present for cingulum rests, especially on mandibular incisors, these rests are most likely to be made with either bonded etched metal or with bonded composite.

A tooth that is contacted by the partial but not through a positive rest cannot be considered an abutment. What might happen in this situation can be illustrated

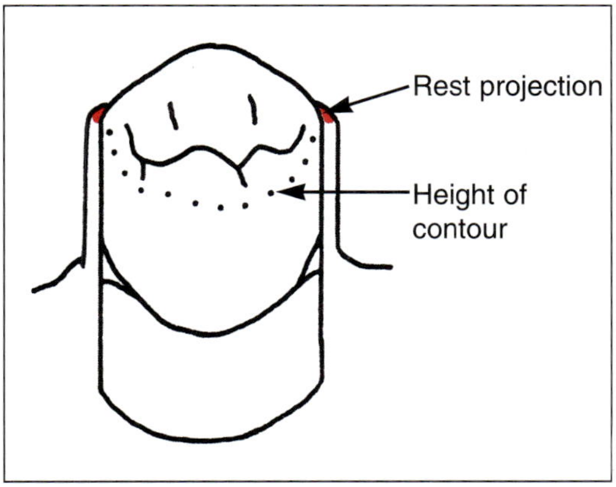

Fig 2-2 Positive rest with guide plates.

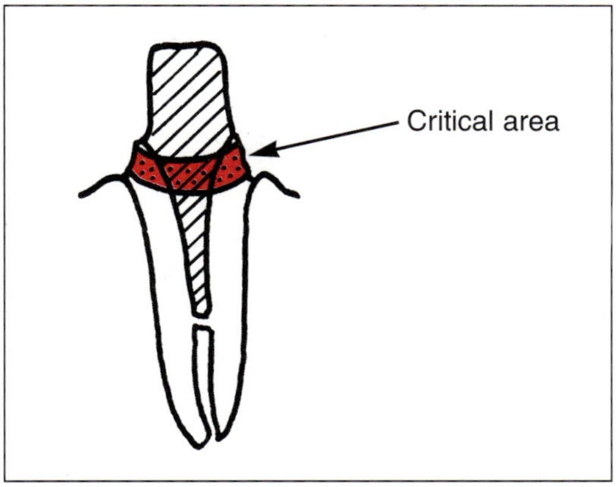

Fig 2-3 Post-core with ferrule (>2 mm).

by a Class I mandibular partial where a lingual plate is used as the major connector; after a period of time, a clinical evaluation shows that the incisors have moved out of contact with the plate. The effect of a positive rest can be obtained with minor connectors (guide plates) alone, but only if they touch the tooth on opposing sides and above the height of contour, since the tooth is then not able to move away from the partial. This situation is rare and usually limited to the management of existing crowns with porcelain occlusal surfaces in cases where preparing an adequate rest may damage a crown that need not otherwise be replaced (Fig 2-2).

A factor that will affect the selection of abutments is the quality of the remaining tooth, both restoratively and periodontally. Crowns must be considered for teeth that have multiple old restorations with marginal leakage. Teeth that are healthy but mobile may need splinting, especially if they are terminal abutments. Teeth that are unlikely to remain for any reason for the expected life of the partial, ie, 10 years, must be extracted before definitive care begins or the framework must be designed with their replacement in mind.

Teeth that are malaligned relative to the plane of occlusion may also be considered compromised abutments and will often require minor tooth movement to make them adequate supports for the partial.

Endodontally compromised teeth that require posts and cores must have adequate tooth structure to allow at least a 2-mm ferrule effect (Fig 2-3). Any previously treated tooth that has had the fill exposed to the oral cavity for any reason must be considered for retreatment before being accepted for use as an abutment.

Connectors

Once the abutments have been selected and the need for restorations (if any) verified, we move on to the second design consideration, that of choosing the connectors, both major and minor. Since the options for the major connectors are arch specific, it is best to consider them independently.

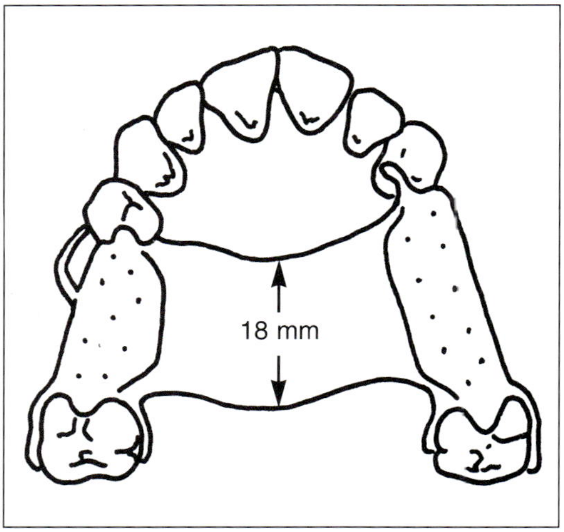

Fig 2-4 Broad palatal strap.

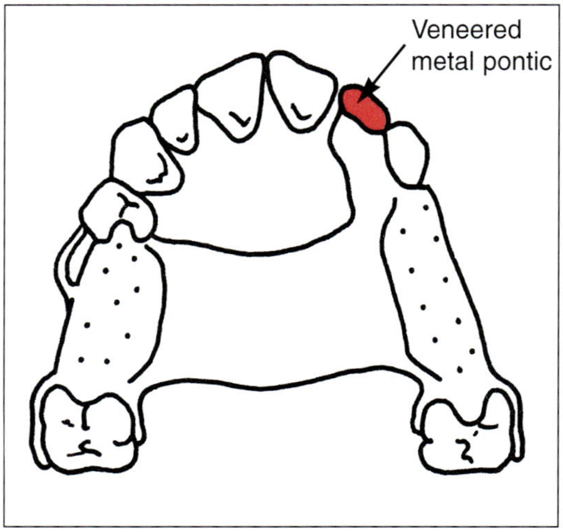

Fig 2-5 Cantilever from palatal strap.

Maxillary Major Connectors

The major connector of choice is one that will, whenever possible, cover neither the anterior nor the posterior palate. Studies have shown that the connector commonly called the "broad palatal strap" is most accepted by patients. This connector crosses the palate in the area of the mesial of the second premolar to the distal of the first molar and must be a minimum of 18 mm to have sufficient rigidity without being too thick (Fig 2-4). A broad palatal strap measuring, for example, 18 mm in width and having a cross-sectional thickness of 0.5 mm will, for all practical purposes, be rigid in normal function. Unless anterior teeth are being replaced by the partial, this design is compatible with all posterior replacement situations. In situations where an isolated lateral incisor is being replaced, the casting can be extended as a cantilever from the canine to keep the anterior palate (speaking area) uncovered (Fig 2-5). In distal extension situations, the major connector is brought posteriorly to flow into the hamular notch area, thus assuring maximum coverage of the edentulous ridge. An alternative design often employed for the maxillae is the anterior-posterior bar, which, I believe, places metal in the least acceptable portion of the palate. The anterior bar will be in the speaking area and the posterior bar will often be too far posterior for patient comfort. The resulting open central palate will have an extended border that can lead to excessive food collection under the partial. Potential further tooth loss within the life of the partial must always be considered in the major connector design, since the teeth in question need to have a lingual plate contact the casting if they are to be added to the partial without affecting the quality of the prosthesis.

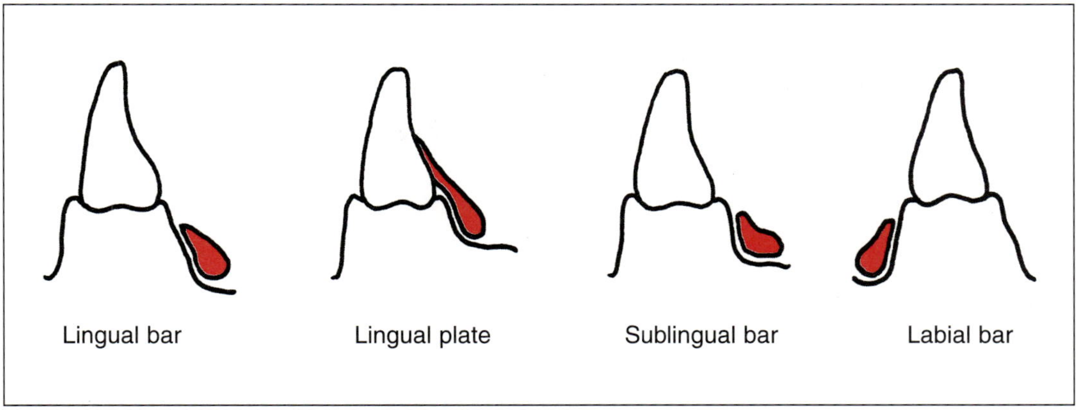

Fig 2-6 Mandibular major connector options.

Mandibular Major Connectors

Selecting a major connector for the mandible should be far easier than for the maxilla. Choices are limited to: lingual bars, sublingual bars, lingual plates, some combination of these three, and, in isolated instances, labial bars. The connector of choice will be that which covers the minimum amount of soft tissue. The standard lingual bar does have space considerations that must be observed. The superior border of the bar must be 3 mm from the gingival margin of the remaining teeth to minimize soft tissue irritation. There must be 4 mm of space for the casting below this point in order to have a rigid major connector with minimum bulk. The commercial clasp patterns used by our laboratories are very close to 4 mm in occlusogingival width. Therefore, 7 mm of space between the gingival marginal tissue of the remaining teeth and the functional depth of the floor of the mouth is essential if a lingual bar is desired. When less space than this is available, the clinician must choose either a lingual plate, where the superior border is at the level of the cingulum and will contact the remaining anterior teeth, or the sublingual bar. The sublingual bar has the same relationship with the gingival tissues of the remaining teeth, but the bar is rotated 90 degrees and placed on the anterior floor of the mouth (Fig 2-6). With this connector, the soft tissues can be left uncovered when 5 mm of space remains in the coverage area. In the few situations where the remaining mandibular teeth are severely lingually inclined, the entire major connector can be brought out into the labial vestibule. The dimensions of the bar must be increased for rigidity since the arc will be longer. The soft tissues are given the same 3-mm clearance as in the lingual bar.

Minor Connectors

In the ideal minor connector relationship, the marginal soft tissues are uncovered whenever possible; 6 mm of clearance from the marginal tissues in the maxilla and 3 mm in the mandible are considered adequate.

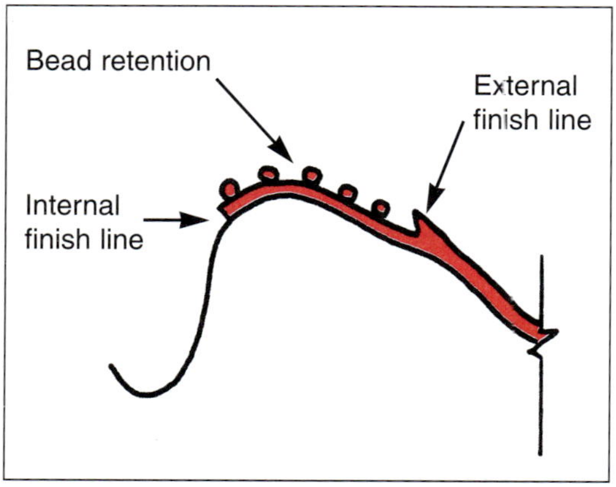

Fig 2-7 Metal base in cross section (maxilla).

The minor connectors are to be placed only onto prepared tooth surfaces. They will take the form of guide plates and rest struts and, where necessary, lingual plates. Numerous studies have shown that soft tissues that are not covered by the partial will be healthier than those that are covered, regardless of the oral hygiene of the patient. Metal dimensions for minor connectors are based primarily on having enough metal present so that the rests will not fracture with time at the marginal ridge. The guide plates can be quite thin (0.5 mm) because they take little or no flexing stress and are not apt to be in occlusal contact. The approach arm of the minor connector must have a minimum of 1.5 mm of metal, both mesiodistally and buccolingually, to ensure adequate strength.

Guiding planes are created whenever possible. They will most likely be found on the proximal surfaces of abutment teeth adjacent to edentulous areas. They can be prepared in the enamel of these abutments or can be added to the tooth in the form of bonded restorations or specially designed crowns. In special situations they are added to lingual surfaces of teeth to isolate the path of insertion/removal. This will most often be done when teeth remain on one side of the arch only, as in maxillary obturators for hemimaxillary resections. The use of multiple guiding planes and the guide plates of the framework that contact them greatly increases the stability and the frictional retention of the RPD.

Resin Retention

The third element of removable partial design is one that is almost always left to the laboratory technician to select, even though it is a decision that is clinically based. For the most part, the choice of retention for the denture teeth and associated base resin is simple. When it is certain that the edentulous area will need to be relined during the life of the partial, then the standard raised mesh is selected. Such situations will be limited to those involving distal extension bases and areas of recent extraction. In every other instance, a metal base with appropriate retentive lugs or loops is indicated. The internal finish line for these metal bases will be a butt joint slightly to the buccal of the ridge crest (Fig 2-7). Metal coverage is preferred because it places highly polished metal over the gingival marginal tissue rather than the thin flash of resin that is commonly found with the standard raised retentive mesh. When mesh must be used, the laboratory must be instructed to use a minimum of one thickness of baseplate wax as the relief pad rather than the usual 24- to 28-gauge wax. The angle of the internal finish line is a critical component of the retentive mechanism. For the raised mesh, the internal line is formed by the shape of the wax relief pad (Fig 2-8). For an ideal internal finish line, the angle formed in the wax must be very

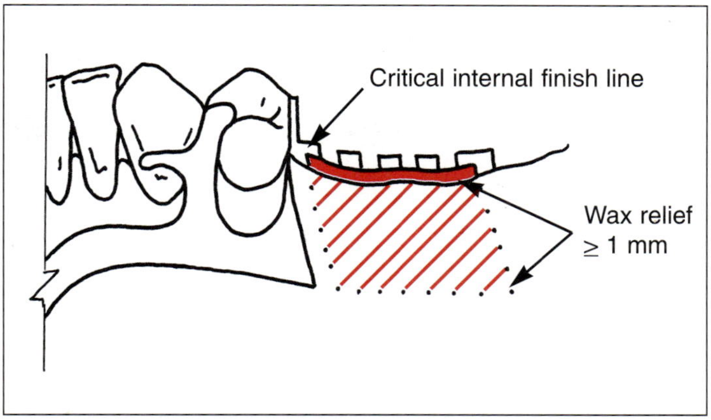

Fig 2-8 Creation of raised mesh.

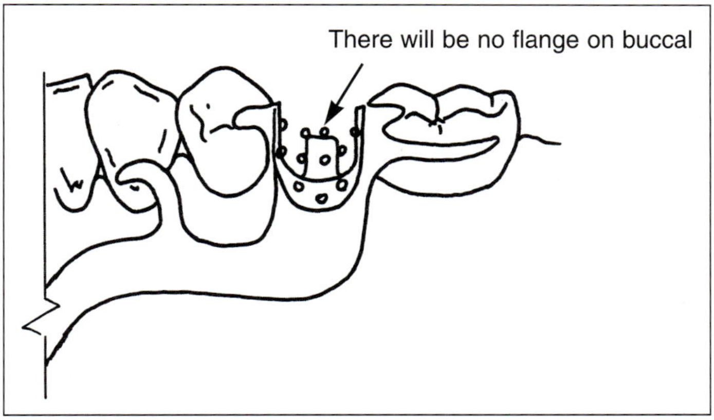

Fig 2-9 Reinforced acrylic pontic for single tooth replacement.

acute so that the resultant contour in the casting will trap the resin in place and reduce the percolation that occurs with thermal changes. Resin bonding agents, properly placed, will overcome the potential for resin-metal separation, but their use is not presently a part of the normal processing protocol in most dental laboratories. The external finish line must also provide an acute angle to lock in the resin and reduce leakage. The finish line must extend from the appropriate line angle to the occlusal surface so that the denture tooth can be placed in a normal position with a small amount of resin between it and the finish line.

For single tooth replacement, there are various options available to the clinician and the technician. Most commonly, some form of reinforced acrylic pontic is chosen. This can be best described as metal ridge coverage with a post extending into the denture tooth. Additional metal beads will enhance the retention (Fig 2-9). Under no circumstances should raised mesh retention be selected for the single tooth, as the amount of retention created in the constricted mesh space is inadequate to retain the denture tooth. When space is lacking, a metal backing, waxed as part of the casting but having the attributes of a fixed pontic, is indicated to provide additional support against the

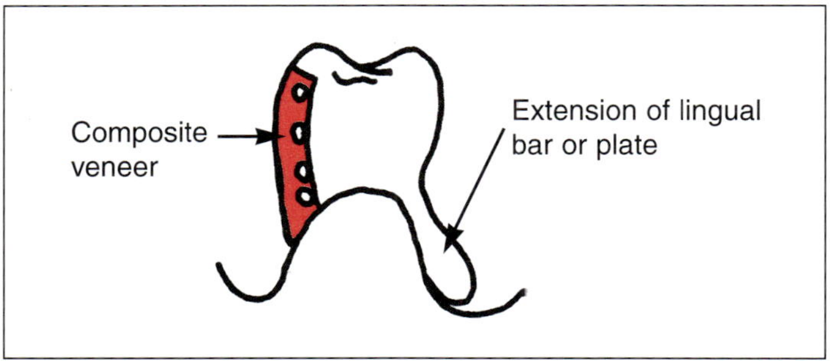

Fig 2-10 Cross section of veneered metal pontic.

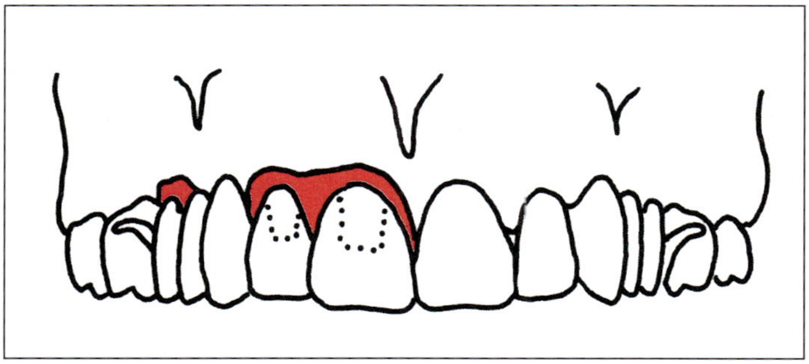

Fig 2-11 Short flange with reinforced acrylic pontics.

forces of incision (Fig 2-10). When the occlusal surface of the pontic is an integral part of the casting, the opposing occlusion, if there is any, must accompany the master cast to the laboratory. When the opposing occlusion is a denture tooth, the anatomy of the occlusal surface of the metal pontic should mimic the selected denture tooth.

The most efficient way to manage the single tooth replacement is to select the denture tooth before the master cast is sent to the lab for the framework. The tooth is ground in to fit the edentulous area, an esthetic try-in is arranged, if appropriate, and a matrix, made of either firm putty or of plaster, is formed to positively position the denture tooth on the master cast. The technician will utilize the matrix and the denture tooth when waxing the framework, and the result will be a retentive form keyed to the ideal tooth position. Obviously, this technique is most often needed for the replacement of anterior teeth and is essential when two or more adjacent anterior teeth are being replaced on the partial. When a denture tooth that matches the shade of the adjacent natural teeth cannot be found, a composite veneer (Visiogem [ESPE, Norristown, PA] or similar material) can be placed in a properly designed metal pontic. These materials can be blended and stained to match almost any tooth. They are, however, quite brittle in shear and, as a result, must have metal at the incisal to protect the veneer. The partial denture casting can be 0.3 mm thick at the incisal or occlusal and still be rigid enough to withstand incising forces. Whenever possible, the single tooth replacement should be planned to exit from the tissue as a fixed pontic, without any resin flange. When two adjacent teeth are replaced, a very short flange may be required to provide for the interdental papilla (Fig 2-11). Often this short flange can be kept very thin and made to closely match the surrounding attached gingiva with minimal tinting of the base when Kayon resin (Kay-See Dental, Kansas City, MO) is used (Earl Pound Technique). For heavily pigmented gingiva, the flange can be packed in clear resin with appropriate tinting so that the patient's gingiva can be seen through the thin flange. The red fibers normally found in standard denture resins must be removed by sifting the polymer through a 2 × 2 gauze since the presence of the fibers in the area of the attached gingiva can never be anatomically correct and will spoil the esthetic effect of even the most carefully tinted resin.

Clasp Retention

The fourth, and final, consideration in the design of the removable partial denture is that of clasp retention. Some clinicians believe that clasp selection is by far the most important consideration in design. However, clasp types, be they I-bar, wire or cast, circumferential or reverse back action, or any of the many others that have found a place in prosthodontics, do not appear to have any clearly defined effect on the clinical success of the partial denture. What is more important is that the clasp be properly made to be strong, retentive, and esthetic, and to do no harm. We will base our selection on these factors alone and will consider the type of clasp to be the least important component of our advanced partial denture.

Since the laboratory plays such a large role in the design of the standard RPD, it is not at all strange that it may emphasize clasp construction. Our technicians are often forced to create castings with little or no evidence of preparation of the remaining teeth. The undesirable undercuts that may exist force the technician to devise ways to work around them, resulting in clasps that are excessive in number and generally unesthetic. A laboratory-designed RPD will usually have more retentive clasps than one designed by a prosthodontist, since careful mouth preparation can be expected to create parallel guiding planes that will give frictional retention. The number of clasps, especially those that might be esthetically unacceptable, can also be reduced by the way the casting is managed when fitting, finishing, and polishing. These techniques will be fully discussed later in this text.

When retentive clasps are contemplated, their length, taper, and cross-sectional width-thickness ratio must be taken into account, as well as the alloy from which they are made and the degree of retentive undercut in which they are placed. All these factors will describe a retentive clasp arm of any configuration that can be expected to function below its proportional limit. Factors that result in distortion of the clasp arm from any cause must be altered so that the clasp will perform as desired for the life of the partial.

Given a mouth that has had ideal mouth preparation, either subtractive or additive, there are only four forms of retentive clasp arms that need be used: *(1)* circumferential cast, *(2)* circumferential wire, *(3)* infrabulge I-bar, and *(4)* infrabulge L-bar.

Circumferential Cast Clasp

This clasp is the most commonly used of all the clasp forms and is easily constructed by the laboratory and adjusted by the clinician. While it is strong, it is also rigid and potentially unesthetic. It is therefore indicated for the posterior part of the mouth and, because of its rigidity, best used in tooth-borne situations.

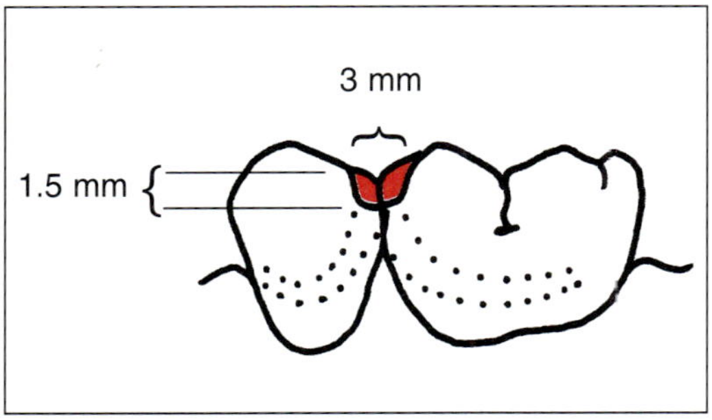

Fig 2-12 Embrasure space for two clasp arms.

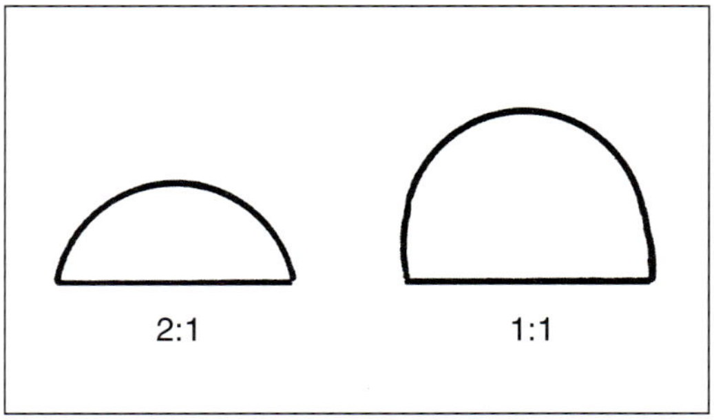

Fig 2-13 Width-thickness ratios for two cast clasp patterns.

A modification of the circumferential clasp commonly found in a variety of situations is the double embrasure clasp, which is nothing but two circumferential clasps back to back. This clasp, used primarily in fully dentate sextants, is unnecessary in conventional RPDs but does have a place in some maxillofacial prostheses. The amount of retention gained from the anterior projecting arms of the embrasure clasp is usually excessive, and when that anterior component is on a premolar, it will become rigid due to its reduced length. The buccal clasp arm is apt to be unesthetic as well. In the well-prepared mouth, the posterior component on the molar provides adequate retention for the conventional partial. The embrasure clasp that passes through a contact area will often break in service because there is seldom enough space created through the contact areas of the two teeth at the embrasure. As a result, the clasp is often found to be in hyperocclusion. Adjusting the metal to allow tooth contact with the opposing arch weakens the clasp by making it thinner at the buccal extension of the marginal ridge than it is further along the clasp arm. This thin area sets up a flexure point in the clasp and, after repeated movement of the clasp arm in function, a stress fracture develops. Repair of this broken embrasure clasp is difficult, if not impossible, to accomplish with any hope of long-term success.

To create adequate space for the most commonly used clasp pattern, the clinician must prepare a channel measuring 1.5 mm by 1.5 mm for one clasp coming through the embrasure and 1.5 mm vertically by 3.0 mm horizontally if two clasps are run through that same embrasure (Fig 2-12). When maximum flexibility is required, a cast circumferential clasp pattern with a width-thickness ratio close to 2:1 (Howmedica pattern 3MA40 is an example) should be requested (Fig 2-13). This might be the case if a cast clasp is used as an embrasure clasp for a Class II mandibular situation where the use of a wrought clasp is not possible. When maximum rigidity and retention is required, as in the case of a maxillary clasp where less than 0.010 inch of retentive area is available in the terminal third at the desired location, then a clasp pattern with a ratio closer to 1:1 would be desirable.

The conventional approach to the cast circumferential clasp requires that a brac-

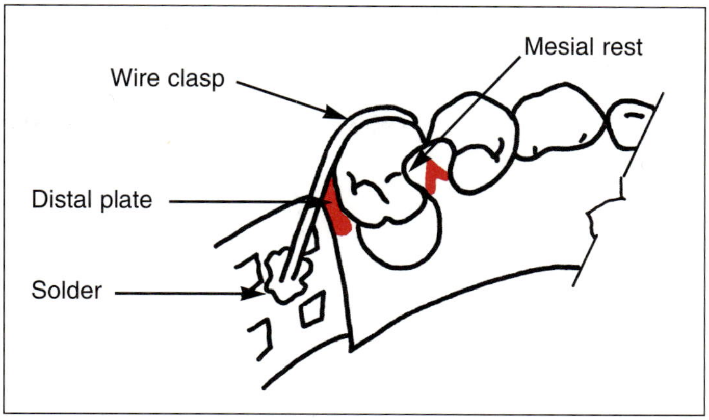

Fig 2-14 Elimination of lingual bracing arm (reciprocation) with guiding planes (red).

ing arm be used to provide reciprocation. This nonflexing arm is traditionally placed as low on the tooth as possible to within 1 mm of the gingiva (that is if the height of contour is at the level of the gingiva, as it may be on the lingual of a maxillary posterior tooth). The need for this bracing arm, customary since the days of banded clasps made of plate gold where both arms entered undercuts, has never been clear to me, especially if the clasp pattern had the same width-thickness ratio as the retentive arm and was of similar length. The ideal bracing arm should be made from a pattern having a width-thickness ratio that approaches 1:1.

There are other ways to achieve reciprocation that are not clasp dependent. These would include precise guiding planes on the minor connectors to the rests as well as the natural contact of the tooth to the adjacent tooth. For the so-called bracing arm to function as it has been proposed it should, it must contact the abutment on a surface parallel to the path of insertion in such a way as to hold the abutment tooth in position as the retentive clasp arm passes over the height of contour and the rest seats fully. This situation normally only occurs when a milled surface has been prepared on a casting for the abutment, since the natural tooth is unlikely to have parallel walls opposite the retentive clasp arm. Once the partial is fully seated, the prepared guiding planes provide lateral bracing in a way that clasp arms never can (Fig 2-14).

Circumferential Wire Clasp

The "wrought wire" clasp, as it is universally known, has long been considered the clasp of choice for Class I and II partial dentures, especially for the mandible. It is obvious that a structure that is cold rolled, as all wires are, is going to be more flexible than a cast clasp of similar dimensions. In addition, because it is round, this clasp will be roughly three times more flexible than a half round cast clasp when loaded other than horizontally, as it would be as the prime retentive element on a mandibular bilateral distal extension partial. The retentive properties of wire are dependent on alloy, length of the active clasp arm, and gauge. The means of attachment of the wire to the framework also has an effect on the flexibility of the clasp; in the most ideal situation, the wire is attached some distance

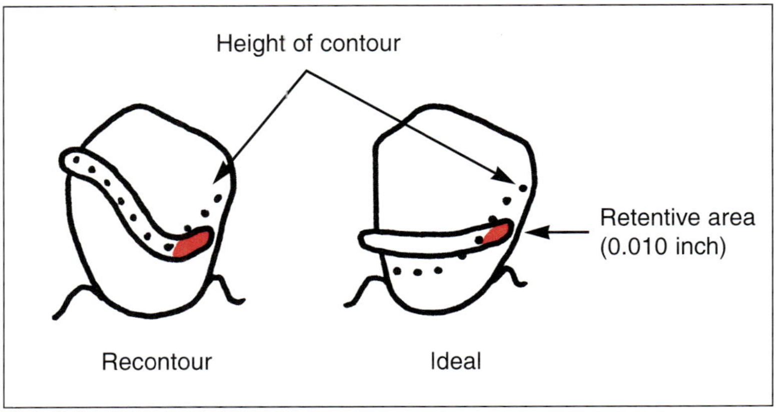

Fig 2-15 Tooth contour for retentive clasps (wire or cast).

from where it is expected to flex. This would normally be on the resin retention area ⅛ inch back from the tooth. Both precious and nonprecious wires can and have been used for retentive clasp arms. There is generally a 1- to 2-gauge difference between a precious wire and one that is an alloy of Ni-Cr or similar material, with the nonprecious wire being stiffer. In fact, both an 18-gauge Ticonium wire (Ni-Cr) and a Baker OR-2 (precious metal) are four times more rigid than a 20-gauge Jelenko Standard wire. An 18-gauge Jelenko wire is two times more rigid than a 20-gauge wire of the same composition. The Jelenko Standard wire has proven to be the alloy of choice (Au 63%, Ag 11%, Pt 10%, Pd 2%, and Cu 13%). Any wire with similar composition could be expected to have similar performance.

To get maximum flexibility from the circumferential wire clasp, every effort must be made to keep the bend placed in the wire in two planes. Historically (and before mouth preparation), wires took the place of plate gold clasps. They were bent to conform to the unmodified tooth contours and, as a result, were bent in the three planes of space, as the clasp made an abrupt bend from the marginal ridge toward the gingival and was then contoured around to the mesial of the tooth to enter the undercut. As each successive bend was made, the wire flexibility was reduced. Accurate tooth modification to reduce the undercuts on the proximal two thirds of the buccal surface allows the clasp to exit from the flange area close to the gingiva and enter the retentive area in the terminal one third to a depth of 0.01 to 0.15 inches (Fig 2-15).

The selection of wires is based primarily on active length according to this simple rule, which allows each wire to perform below its proportional limit: Clasps with an active length < 7 mm should be of 20-gauge, those 8 to 10 mm should be of 19-gauge, and those > 10 mm will require an 18-gauge wire. At these distances and these gauges, the wires will give approximately

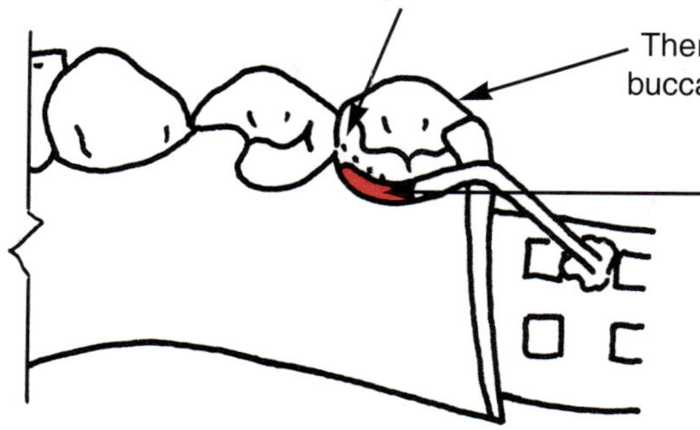

Fig 2-16 Lingual retentive wire clasp above lingual plate.

the same amount of retention and remain below their proportional limit. While it may be possible to place some wires into undercuts > 0.15 inch and still have them function without distortion, there is no clinical evidence that this increase in undercut depth is of any value. The wire clasp can be used successfully on the lingual surface of most mandibular premolars, in conjunction with a distal guide plate that extends slightly beyond the distal facial line angle and a mesial rest, to provide retention without any display of buccal metal. In these situations, the clasp arm will be very short and must therefore be of 20-gauge or finer wire. The major connector must be a lingual or sublingual bar, at least in the area of this clasp, so that the requirement for 3 mm of space at the superior margin of the bar is essential. In the maxilla, the major connector is opened to the lingual as a matter of course whenever possible, so that finding a lingual surface for the wire retentive clasp arm is not normally a problem if the tooth contours provide any retentive areas of 0.010 inch or greater. There is no need for a buccal bracing arm in these situations. When the major connector cannot be opened for any reason, it is still possible to utilize only a lingual clasp arm if sufficient tooth height exists to permit the wire to sit on the occlusal border of the lingual plate and enter the proper undercut. The only disadvantage to this design is the slight opening of the major connector beneath the clasp tip (Fig 2-16).

Unlike cast clasp arms that can be expected to break if they are deformed and then recontoured more than a few times, wire clasps (especially those of high-gold alloys) will withstand repeated readaptation without any change in their retentive properties. Since these clasps are more flexible, they have the disadvantage of being far easier for the patient to deform if they are used as handles to remove the partial from the mouth. Patients must be warned that deformation of a properly

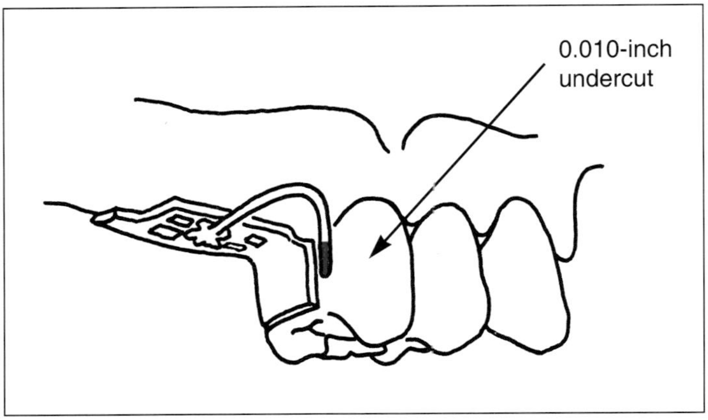

Fig 2-17 Short wire I-bar to distobuccal retentive area.

placed wire clasp can only occur if the wire is loaded beyond its proportional limit and that this can happen only if the clasp is distorted by the patient. Some patients insist on biting their partials to place rather than placing them with the fingers of both hands. Patients must be shown that they can use the flanges of the denture base as a purchase point for removing the denture. Sometimes the placement of a simulated Class V cavity on a denture tooth will give the patient a purchase point to apply a dislodging force.

Infrabulge Clasps

Infrabulge clasps have long been advocated as an alternative to the wire circumferential clasp for Class I and II situations. They have been proposed as a more esthetic alternative to the cast circumferential clasp as well. These clasps can come in a number of forms and can be either cast or wrought. The most commonly used infrabulge clasp has been the I-bar, which is to be placed at the greatest convexity of the tooth mesiodistally as seen from the horizontal. When combined with a proximal guide plate at the edentulous side of the prime abutment and a rest at the other end of the occlusal surface, no bracing arm is required. This is because the tooth cannot be displaced by the action of the retentive clasp arm. Depending on the contact of the guide plate, stress relief can be created with this system for the Class I situation.

When the I-bar clasp is made of a suitable length and gauge of wire, additional advantages are possible. Since the wire is added to the casting by soldering after the frame has been finished and polished, it is possible to place the clasp arm very close to the buccal extension of the guide plate (Fig 2-17). With this distal positioning, the clasp arm becomes shorter and must therefore be of a higher gauge to retain flexibility (normally a 20-gauge wire will be chosen). The guiding plane and plate must extend fully to the line angle, and a positive rest on the opposite side of the abutment must be used to provide reciprocation if the distally placed I-bar is on a terminal abutment. If this type of clasping is used on the anterior abutment of a Class III partial denture, the need for precise reciprocation is not as great because the posterior abutment will restrict distal movement of the partial.

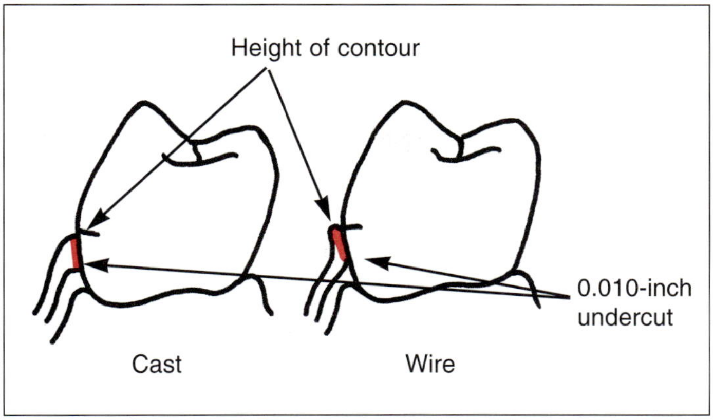

Fig 2-18 Tooth–bar clasp relationship.

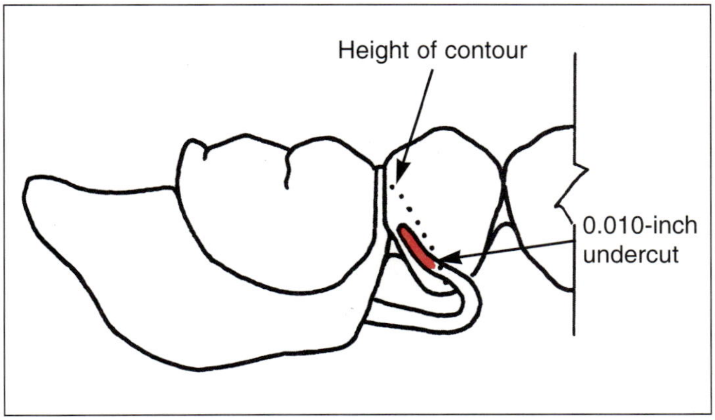

Fig 2-19 Contour indicating the need for L-bar clasp.

The contact between the I-bar and the retentive area must not be a point contact. Instead, the wire is contoured in such a way as to present a line contact or a surface contact. When a cast I-bar is used, the surface contact is created in the blockout and waxing of the framework (Fig 2-18). These expanded contact areas provide a margin of error for the technician, since placing a clasp tip at point contact on a repeated basis is an unreasonable request.

While the I-bar clasp is by far the most common of the infrabulge clasps, there is an occasional need for an L-bar when the only available usable undercut is immediately adjacent to the edentulous area and where even a light-wire I-bar will be too short and therefore too rigid. By bringing the approach arm up to the midbuccal of the tooth and then bringing the base of the L distally to the retentive area, sufficient clasp length can be developed in most situations (Fig 2-19). This clasp form can be created in either cast metal or with wire, again remembering to choose the appropriate gauge based on the active length of the clasp.

Other forms of bar clasps have been advocated over the years, primarily the T-bar and occasionally a U-bar. These forms have no place in the modern RPD and are generally unesthetic and difficult, if not impossible, to adjust—especially if they are made in cast metal.

There is one major contraindication for the infrabulge clasp. The height of contour of the soft tissue in the area of the proximal approach arm and the degree of soft tissue undercut can make the bar clasps unacceptable. If the height of contour is very close to the buccal marginal tissue, the approach arm will have to stand out from the tissue because it cannot be in an undercut relative to the path of insertion as determined by the guiding planes. If that soft tissue undercut is severe, the clasp may abrade the buccal mucosa in normal function.

Even the most casual glance at any text on removable partial dentures will identify many other clasp forms: ring clasps, back action clasps, "C" or fish hook clasps, and on and on. These clasp forms have all been created to work around contours that have not been adequately modified with appropriate mouth preparation or, in some cases, teeth that need minor orthodontia to return them to a normal position in the arch. If there is no usable mesial undercut for a circumferential wire clasp, undercuts on the lingual surface will have to be used or the tooth modified with some form of additive mouth preparation. Given quality mouth preparation, no other clasp forms, beyond the cast and wrought circumferential clasps and the I-bar and L-bar clasps, either wrought or cast, are indicated.

There are two other general categories of cast retentive elements that will be considered later (Chapter 9): the rotational path of insertion partial and the hinged connector (commonly referred to as a "Swinglock"). These two special types of frameworks may include conventional clasping in addition to their special retentive devices.

Design Specifics: Class I–IV

With an understanding of the component parts of the partial denture, we can now look to specific design considerations for each of the four basic classifications of the RPD. There will be many areas of overlap in design, but the intent of this section is to identify basic principles of design for each class independently, keeping in mind the four component parts of partial denture therapy.

Before any specific designs can be established, a quality diagnostic cast must be available for surveying. The cast must accurately represent all remaining teeth and those soft tissue–covered areas that will be within the denture space. This would include retromolar pads, frenum extensions, vestibules when bar clasps are being considered, and the like.

Finding the Path of Insertion

The first step will always be to determine the path of insertion and removal. Here the emphasis is on the path of removal, since the goal will be to limit the possible directions that the partial can exit from the mouth through preparation of hard tissues. The path of insertion is, of course, the reciprocal of the more important path of removal and is most often presented as being of some importance. In all but one instance, the path of removal should be parallel to the long axis of the prime abutment(s). There will be occasions, usually in Class IV situations and especially in those where a rotational path of insertion is planned, when the path of removal is primarily determined by the soft tissue height of contour.

The path of insertion/removal is frozen in space by the prepared guiding planes and the cast plates that touch them. Undercuts on hard or soft tissue exist only relative to that path, so tilting the cast on the surveyor in order to alter the relative heights of contour to obtain retention will not produce real undercuts unless the path is controlled by the planes. Given the frictional retention that parallel guide plates can provide, there is seldom any need to be concerned about retention. If there are no usable retentive areas anywhere on the desired abutment teeth, then they must be created by either subtractive or additive mouth preparation.

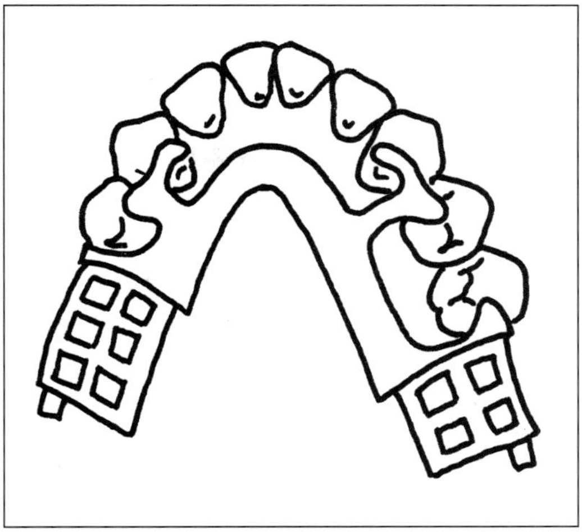

Fig 2-20 Multiple abutments are used when possible.

Class I RPD

Abutment Selection and Rests

Only when the canine is the prime abutment (ie, the abutment adjacent to the distal extension base) should a single abutment be chosen for the Class I partial. A first premolar used by itself as the only abutment does not provide sufficient support to replace the missing molars and the second premolar. When the first premolar is the prime abutment, it must have an occlusal rest and the adjacent canine must have either a distal-incisal or a cingulum rest (for the mandible, this rest cannot be made deep enough and kept in enamel, so either bonded metal or bonded composite must be used to create the rest seat). When both premolars remain, their bony support must be evaluated. If they have excellent bone levels and the opposing arch is a complete denture, the canine rest may be eliminated, leaving the two premolars as the abutments. Since it is rare to replace only a second molar on a Class I RPD, the only options we need concern ourselves with are those just mentioned. The Class I RPD will have a single abutment if the abutment tooth is the canine, and two abutments if the first premolar is the prime abutment. If the second premolar is the prime abutment, then there will be either two or three abutments, based on the level of bony support (Fig 2-20). The position of the occlusal rests on the premolars is immaterial, although some would say that a mesial rest on the prime abutment is superior to a distal rest. While there may well be theoretical differences here, there appears to be no difference clinically in the well-made and maintained RPD. The path of insertion/removal will be chosen to allow parallelism of the distal surfaces of the prime abutments.

The guiding planes created on the prime abutments require a basic decision regarding stress relief. Two techniques have been proposed over the years. Kratochvil suggested that the guiding plane be prepared to be as long as possible, with the stress relief coming from a functional relief of the

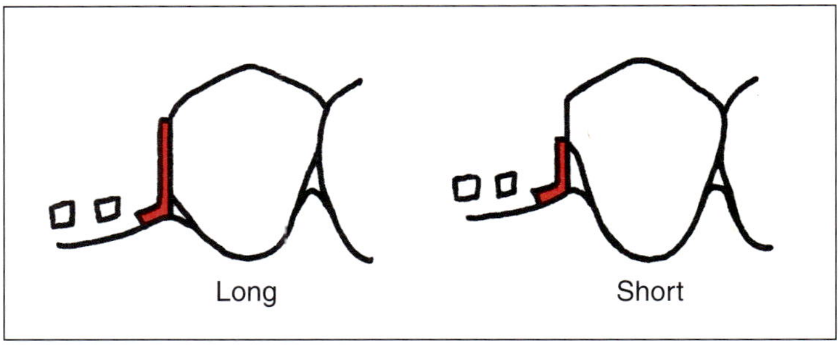

Fig 2-21 Guiding plane/guide plate options for Class I partials.

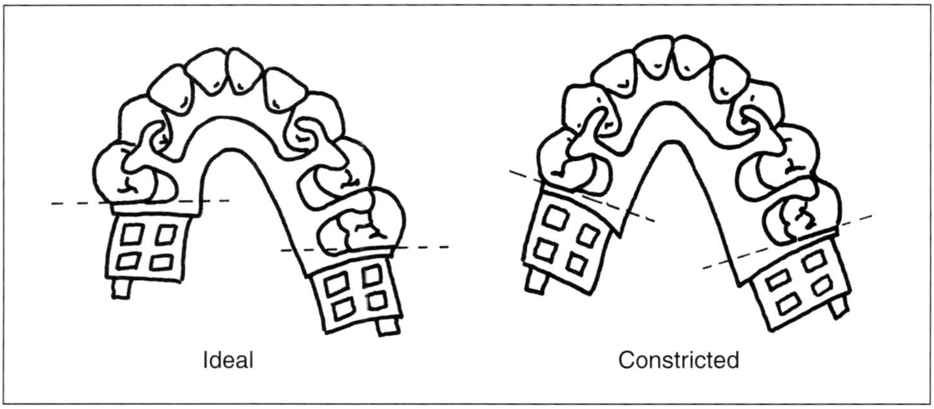

Fig 2-22 Ideal parallism of guiding planes to allow unrestricted rotation.

casting before the altered cast impression was made. Kroll, on the other hand, described a shorter guiding plane extending from the marginal ridge roughly one third of the way down the tooth, with the occlusal limit of the guide plate being the gingival extension of this shorter guiding plane (Fig 2-21). Here, the stress relief is created in the blockout of the undercut gingival to the guiding plane. The guide plate is effective in reciprocation but can also rotate into the undercut rather than bind on the guiding plane during loading of the posterior denture bases. There is no clinical evidence that would favor one of these approaches over the other. The decision may well rest on the quality of the laboratory support, since the reduced-length guiding plane/guide plate requires greater attention to detail in both blockout and finishing of the casting.

In either approach, the parallel guiding planes, contacted by the guide plates of the casting, restrict the path of insertion/removal to whatever angle of divergence was established in the mouth preparation phase of the treatment. The closer to 90 degrees parallelism, the greater the frictional resistance to dislodgment with the potential for stress relief still viable. For the Class I partial denture, parallelism must be considered in another plane of space. In order for the partial to rotate freely around its fulcrum, the guiding planes must be parallel to each other from the occlusal view as they are in the sagittal. That is, they must lie on the same plane across the arch so they can act in an identical fashion under occlusal load (Fig 2-22). For any of the other classes, the effect of the planes is enhanced by being in different planes as seen from the occlusal.

The same considerations exist for the opposite side of the mouth, with the only compromise coming when the distal slopes of the two prime abutments are not parallel and cannot be made so through subtractive mouth preparation. When this occurs (usually when the canines are prime abutments), the best option is to favor the weaker of the two prime abutments. The other (stronger) abutment will be recontoured with additive mouth preparation to allow both sides to be parallel.

Connectors

As stated before, whenever possible, the maximum amount of soft tissue should remain uncovered by the RPD. This would require, for example, the use of the lingual bar over the lingual plate. If, however, there is inadequate space or if there is the potential for loss of some remaining anterior teeth during the life of the partial, a lingual plate will be the proper choice so that additions can be made successfully. It may be possible to combine a lingual plate in the incisor area with a lingual bar distal to the canines instead of covering all the lingual surfaces. When space permits, this design is preferred because it offers the potential for lingual retentive clasping and no show of metal on the buccal surfaces of the abutments.

The maxillary Class I major connector varies in the placement of both the anterior and the posterior borders. As the number of teeth to be replaced with the partial increases, the natural inclination will be to in-

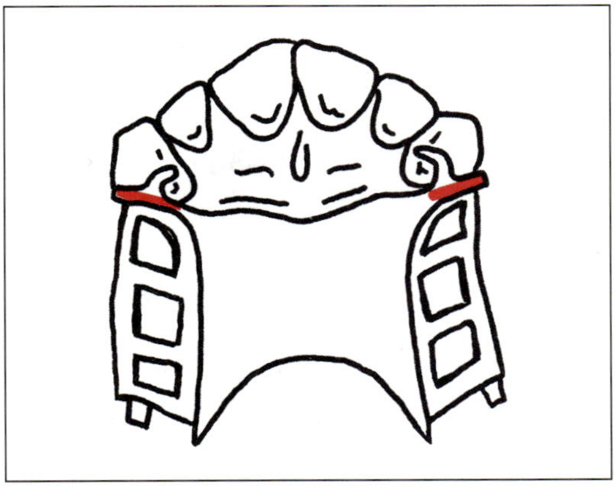

Fig 2-23 Minimal coverage of anterior palate requires large guiding planes for positive results.

crease the coverage of the major connector so that it approaches a complete denture outline. Since there can be no peripheral seal on the partial denture, there is little value in extending the posterior border to the vibrating line. The glandular portion of the posterior soft palate offers no real support to the partial, and therefore should be left uncovered. The edentulous ridges, however, do support the partial and should always be covered to the hamular notch, either in resin or with metal. Anterior coverage is dependent on the teeth remaining. If only the six anteriors are left, going to full lingual coverage offers the option of easy addition of teeth should some be lost, as well as providing the potential for additional frictional retention on any guiding planes that can be established. Finding tooth structure on the lingual of maxillary anterior teeth that can be prepared to parallel guiding surfaces is, unfortunately, uncommon. When the remaining six anterior teeth are healthy and not mobile, it is certainly feasible to open the anterior area by projecting a cingulum rest onto a prepared acute rest preparation from the distal. The anterior border must then blend into the anterior slope of the rugae area and end posterior to a major rugae. For this approach to be dependably successful, the canines must have sufficient distal structure to allow for guiding planes of at least 3 mm (Fig 2-23).

Minor connectors will be of standard dimensions, with care taken to see that at least 1.2 mm of metal thickness at the marginal ridge is available to support the rests.

Resin Retention

Since the need for periodic reline of the distal extension base is expected, especially on the mandibular arch, the resin retention of choice is a raised mesh with > 1 mm of space for resin below the mesh. In some situations on the maxilla, where there has been minimal resorption of the edentulous extension (and therefore minimal room for the casting and the replacement denture teeth), a metal base with retentive beads as an intregal part of the casting is the only viable option. Obviously, this base cannot be relined; however, in the mature edentulous ridge with the support of the palatal coverage, no reline may be needed during the life of the partial.

Modification spaces are managed with metal bases and bead or post retention wherever possible. Only very recent extractions could be considered for mesh retention, but caution must be taken for a single tooth replacement because the amount of mesh retention available for the single tooth is often inadequate. It is generally wiser to add a tooth to the existing partial denture temporarily, or to construct an interim partial for the initial healing period and then construct the new RPD with either a reinforced metal post or a veneered pontic form for the single tooth.

Clasping

The type of retentive clasp to be used is determined by two factors: the availability of a retentive area on the tooth and the clinician's preference. The options may be classified as follows:

- Only a mesiobuccal retentive area—wire circumferential clasp to 0.015 inch.
- Midfacial retentive area with appropriate gingival contour—I-bar to 0.010 inch (either cast or wrought).
- Only a distofacial retentive area—L-bar to 0.010 inch (preferably wrought).
- No facial retentive areas are present—lingual wire circumferential clasps to 0.010 inch or recontour abutment with either subtractive or additive preparation.

In either arch, one retentive clasp per side will provide adequate retention if the maximum frictional retention is established through mouth preparation and careful fitting of the casting.

In choosing the retentive clasps for the mandibular Class I RPD, consideration must be given to establishing stress relief because the partial will always rotate in function. The maxillary RPD may show very little rotational movement due to the support of the hard palate and the generally superior ridge contour. The weaker the abutment teeth and the supporting ridge, the greater the rotational movement that must be allowed in the fit of the casting. This relief can be obtained in the blockout of the master cast or in the intraoral fitting of the frame (to be discussed later). Along with the fit of the frame, the flexibility of the retentive clasp arms selected plays an important role in stress relief, so that a light-wire retentive clasp in any of the appropriate clasp

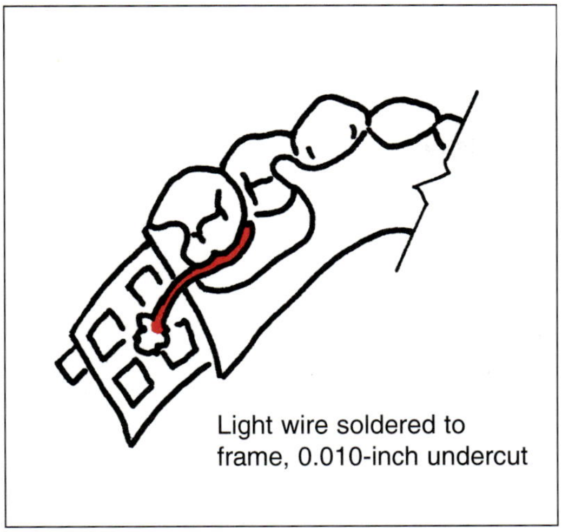

Fig 2-24 Elimination of buccal bracing arm with lingual retentive wire.

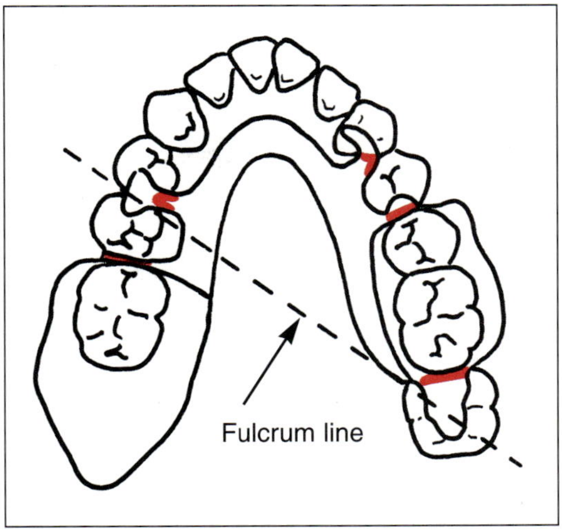

Fig 2-25 Guiding planes restricting rotation in the Class II partial.

forms is indicated when the support is poor. This decision may sacrifice some retention and stability to relieve the abutment teeth from the full load of mastication.

In the Class I RPD, there is no need to consider the use of a so-called "bracing clasp" because the combination of rests/minor connectors and guide plates and tooth contacts will provide the necessary reciprocation. Even if lingual circumferential clasping is chosen, it is not necessary to complicate the casting and show unsightly metal with a buccal bracing clasp arm (Fig 2-24).

Class II RPD

Abutments and Rests

While the Class II partial design is often considered a mixture of the principles of Class I and Class III partial designs, special consideration must be given to the potential for rotation at the fulcrum line that will run from the distalmost rigid contacts of the partial with the abutment teeth on each side of the arch. One might imagine that rotation and the resulting stress relief will occur naturally without any effort. In truth, a decision as to the desirability of allowing motion around the fulcrum line must be made before mouth preparation begins. For the most part, there is no need to plan for stress relief for the Class II RPD because the remaining teeth, if properly contacted on prepared surfaces (and in particular on guiding plane surfaces), will be able to support the teeth being replaced as a cantilever (Fig 2-25). Mastication will most often occur on the dentate (Class II) side due to increased efficiency in managing food particles, so the distal extension side will receive only minor loading. Only when the abutments are weak and few in number must we consider reducing the length of the guiding planes and functional relief of the casting to allow limited rotation and partial loading of the edentulous ridge. When the casting has been relieved, the support of the edentulous area is obtained through the altered cast impression. In the maxillary arch,

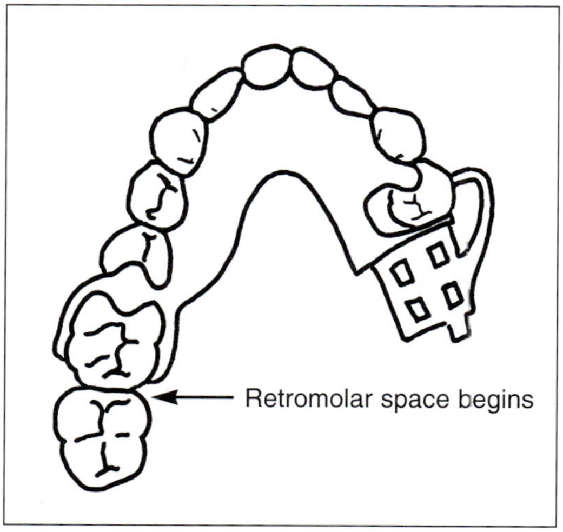

Fig 2-26 Stopping major connector short of retromolar space.

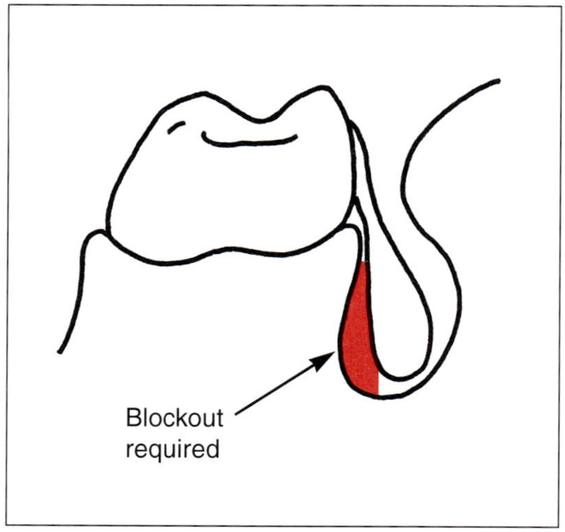

Fig 2-27 Major connector forced to stand away from tissue in retromolar space.

additional support for the weakened teeth is obtained by covering a greater portion of the palate, and an altered cast impression is normally not needed.

The distal extension side of the partial is treated exactly as in the Class I situation with no exceptions. The management of the tooth-supported side offers a few options usually dependent on the number, strength, and position of the available abutments. When the dentate side is complete, ie, no modification spaces, an embrasure clasp on the first molar is the retention of choice. This clasp must be cast, since the construction of an embrasure clasp made of wire is technically very difficult and the long-term dependability of such a clasp very much in question. The embrasure clasp is placed on the first molar rather than the second because the mandible curves into the retromolar space starting at about the second molar, which requires that the major connector going back to a second molar stand far away from the tissue, creating a food trap that patients do not appreciate (Figs 2-26 and 2-27). The first molar is more apt to allow the placement of the major connector in a comfortable position. Under no circumstances should a premolar be used in place of the molar, since any clasp placed on it will be shorter and more rigid and often unesthetic as well.

The need for additional abutments on the tooth-borne side must be considered. At the very minimum, an additional minor connector and rest must be placed as far forward from the embrasure clasp as possible. This rest/connector combination has been called an indirect retainer, and it was assumed that it would counteract the upward rotation of the edentulous base. This antirotation device springs from dentistry's past, as far as partial denture design is concerned, when no mouth preparation for guiding planes was done. In the modern RPD, the guiding planes and the intimate contact with the casting through the guide plates prohibits rotation until the partial has moved beyond the contact of the guiding plane and the associated guide plate. Only at that point can the denture rotate and the "indirect retainer" come into antirotational contact. So, while

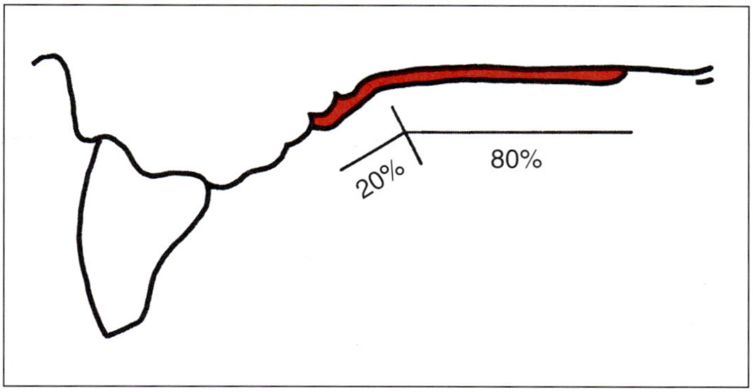

Fig 2-28 Configuration of broad palatal strap in cross section.

true indirect retention is a thing of the past, the use of an additional rest/minor connector some distance from the embrasure clasp is essential to provide a third point of reference for seating the framework during fitting of the frame, making the altered cast impression, and re-relating the framework during future relines of the distal extension base.

The mesial of the mandibular first premolar and the distal of the maxillary first premolar are often used for this third point of contact. The mesial of the mandibular first premolar is ideal from a geometric standpoint, but, unfortunately, the amount of tooth structure at the marginal ridge may not allow the preparation of an ideal, acute occlusal rest. The mesial of the maxillary first premolar would also be ideal, but disclusion often occurs at the contact of the premolar and the canine, limiting the available space for minor connector and rest.

When a modification space(s) is present, we have the potential to develop additional frictional retention and reciprocation by maximizing the guiding plane surfaces adjacent to the edentulous space(s) through either subtractive or additive tooth preparation. At the very minimum, a rest and guiding plane would be placed on the isolated molar abutment and the tooth at the anterior extension of the edentulous space. Additional abutments would be added as required if the support from the two original abutments appeared to be inadequate.

Guiding planes for the Class II partial denture should be as long as possible, provided that the casting is planned as a cantilever. If stress relief is indicated, the casting will be adjusted intraorally.

Connectors

Major and minor connector design on the dentate side of the partial, in both the maxilla and the mandible, will be that of the Class III RPD. Every attempt is made to cover as little gingival tissue as possible. The dimensions of the castings and their relation to the soft tissues are the same as for the Class I situation, while the third point of contact (indirect retainer) in the maxilla may require the major connector to be moved toward the anterior. The minor connector to that rest must blend into the rugae area of the maxilla so that the speaking area is not compromised. Placing a small part (one fifth) of the major connector onto the slope of the anterior palate and the remaining four fifths on the more posterior horizontal palate will strengthen the casting, as the corrugation in the metal allows for a thinner casting with the same rigidity (Fig 2-28).

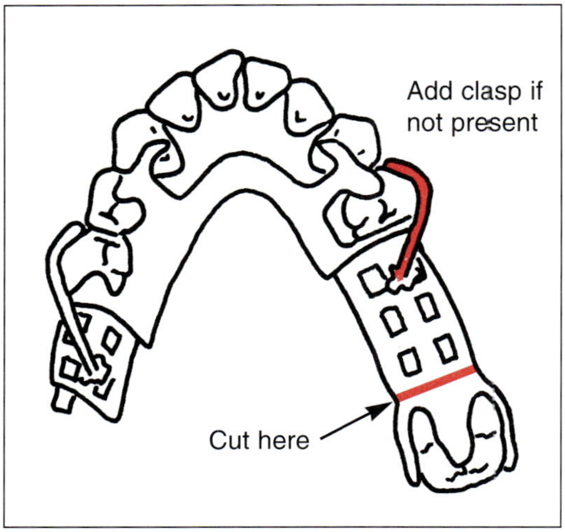

Fig 2-29 Conversion of Class II to Class I with loss of molar.

Modification spaces for missing anterior teeth present a special problem in that they complicate the design of the casting and often require that metal be placed in the speaking area of the anterior palate. When a lateral incisor is missing, it may be possible to cantilever it off the rest and minor connector on the canine, but when central and lateral or two central incisors are missing, a full anterior casting will be required. A better solution to this problem is to replace missing anterior teeth with fixed or bonded partial dentures and leave the RPD to replace only posterior teeth.

Resin Retention

The resin retention for the tooth-borne side of the Class II RPD favors the use of metal coverage of the ridge whenever possible, according to requirements mentioned earlier. If only a single tooth is being replaced, special consideration must be given to metal retention because the space is often restricted. Usually some form of a retentive post is designed to fall within the denture tooth. When the desired tooth position is obvious, then the post can be randomly placed by the technician. When the tooth needs to be in some irregular position due to esthetic requirements or abnormal occlusal relations, then the denture tooth must be ground into place by the clinician, verified in the patient's mouth, and sent along with the master cast in some sort of matrix so that the technician knows exactly where the tooth must be placed.

A final consideration for the Class II mandibular RPD is the potential for conversion after additional tooth loss. The isolated posterior abutment on the tooth-borne side is often a weakened tooth, both restoratively and periodontally, and may not last the life of the partial. In anticipation of the loss of this tooth, the partial should be designed as if it were a Class I RPD, with raised retentive mesh, a mesial rest on the premolar that would become the prime abutment on that side of the arch, and with the potential for flexible clasping on the prime abutment. In addition, the internal and external finishing lines must be positioned as if the posterior abutment did not exist, ie, at the distolingual of the premolar that will become the prime abutment. The retentive mesh, suitably reinforced, then runs distally to the isolated molar and its clasp assembly (Fig 2-29). When the molar is lost, the rest, clasp, and guide plate are cut off and the resin base is extended to cover the total denture space during reline/rebase procedures.

Unfortunately, the maxillary arch cannot be treated in the same fashion for conversion since the major connector in the maxilla will not have a finish line assembly that can be converted to a Class I. Attempts to solder on finishing lines and associated meshwork are technically very complicated, and the cost seldom justifies the conversion.

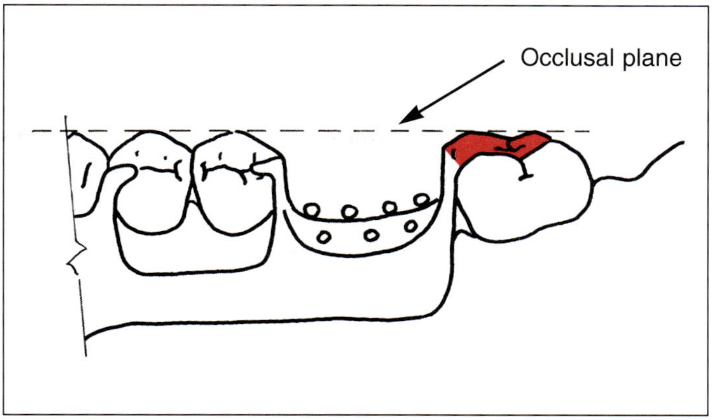

Fig 2-30 Long onlay rest on molar restores occlusal plane for opposing complete denture.

Clasping

Again, the clasp requirements for the distal extension side of the Class II are identical to those of the Class I. On the tooth-borne side, there is a major decision to be made. Since it is rare to find a mandibular situation where more than one clasp per side is needed for retention, the clinician must choose between clasping on the fulcrum line or anterior to it. In most cases, the posterior abutment on the tooth-borne side will be a molar, since if it were a premolar the case would be considered a Class I. The advantages are clearly on the side of clasping on the fulcrum line, ie, the molar on the tooth-borne side and the terminal abutment on the other side. Clasp selection for the molar is generally limited to a circumferential clasp, either cast or wire, with the lingual arm being retentive. This is because the retentive area is most apt to be found on that side of the tooth due to its natural inclination in the arch. Since this clasp will be the terminal of the RPD, some reciprocation will be required to maintain the tooth in the arch and prevent it from moving away from the partial. This can be done in two ways: *(1)* with a conventional guide plate/rest and bracing arm combination or *(2)* with the use of an extended guide plate (one that extends slightly from the mesial to the buccal and lingual surfaces) combined with an oversized occlusal rest that extends to the distal fossa. This long rest has the additional advantage of allowing the restoration of the plane of occlusion with the rest if the distal abutment has indeed migrated mesially and lingually (Fig 2-30).

If the molar is so severely tilted that the retentive area is very deep and very near the occlusal surface, with minor orthodontics not an option for whatever reason, it may be best not to clasp that tooth. Instead, consideration should be given to retaining the guiding plane and the extended occlusal rest and moving the retentive clasp anterior to the fulcrum (to the premolar). The clasp choice in this situation can be either a circumferential clasp or an infrabulge clasp. The retentive arm will be anterior to the fulcrum, so a wire circumferential clasp arm is selected over a cast one because the potential for greater movement of the partial in function in that area dictates a more flexible clasp. As in other esthetic areas, a wire I-bar clasp, set to the distal, may be the best choice.

In the maxilla, a case can be made for the use of three retentive clasps if a modification space exists on the dentate side, since the force of gravity adds another dimension to the retentive requirement. Here, the molar clasp will most likely be a cast circumferential and the clasp on the distal extension side an I-bar, since this clasp is less likely to be visible when the patient smiles and speaks. The I-bar clasp has been presented as having to be placed midway on the tooth mesiodistally in order to function with minimum stress on the abutment. While this may be true in the mandible, there is not enough movement possible on a well-fitting maxillary casting to make any clinical difference. For this reason, the I-bar clasp can be set as far to the distal as possible as long as there is a mesial rest and a distal guide plate. If a wire I-bar is used, it is possible to place the clasp almost in contact with the buccal extension of the guide plate because this clasp is added to the framework after the frame has been finished and polished. A cast infrabulge clasp must be placed farther from the guide plate so that space is available to finish and polish the clasp, making the clasp potentially more visible on the tooth. The third clasp, placed on the anterior abutment on the tooth-supported side, should also be a wire I-bar clasp for the reasons given. If no modification space exists, there will be an increased reliance on the creation of multiple guiding planes to restrict the movement of the partial denture.

Class III RPD

This classification of partial denture could really be called a "removable fixed bridge." In most situations, it uses the same abutments as would a fixed partial denture replacing the same missing teeth. The design options, at first glance, might appear to be endless, but in truth can be reduced to only a few basic options as long as the clinician is willing to prepare the mouth ideally. Four obvious treatment considerations govern the choice of the removable partial denture in the Class III situation over a fixed partial denture. The first and most influential reason is cost. The second relates to those situations where the length of span of the edentulous area and the periodontal support of the remaining possible abutment teeth combine to bring into question the long-term success of a fixed partial denture. The third reason is strictly one of esthetics. There are instances when the need to replace the interdental papillae in the anterior of the mouth make the fixed partial denture unacceptable. While it is true that ridge augmentation in any of its many forms can create an adequate gingival base, the restoration of the papillae is not always possible. Last, there will always be those situations where the loss of teeth was accompanied by traumatic loss of the alveolar process as well. In these cases, the need to replace missing soft tissue requires the use of a flange of such dimensions that the appliance be removable to allow the patient access for proper hygiene. The goal of removable partial denture treatment for the Class III patient must be to make the appliance conform to the principles of fixed partial dentures as much as possible.

Abutment Selection

The choice of abutments is generally obvious: one abutment on each end of an edentulous area. This general statement is mod-

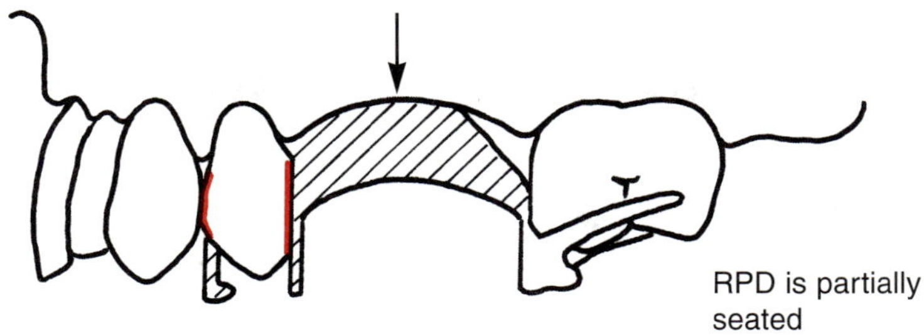

Fig 2-31 Anterior guiding planes preclude rotation away from tissue.

ified by adding abutments when the potential support of the teeth is in question. Whenever this question arises, it is better to add another abutment because additional frictional retention can be obtained. Unlike the case of the fixed partial denture, in which splinted abutments bring potential problems of embrasure access and connector rigidity, double-abutting in the removable partial situation causes no particular problems. Remember, abutments must have positive rest preparations to maintain contact between the partial and teeth over the life of the partial. These ideal rest shapes can usually be created with subtractive mouth preparation in the posterior of the mouth, but additive mouth preparation is often required for the anterior teeth.

In addition to selecting the abutments and planning their rests, the potential for parallel guiding planes must be evaluated through careful consideration of the path of insertion/removal. The goal of the mouth preparation for the Class III case is to maximize the frictional retention of the guiding planes/guide plates to totally eliminate the need for any anterior clasping. Posterior clasping, one clasp on each side, is more than sufficient when the anterior portion of the partial is controlled by the guiding planes. This partial denture cannot rotate out of the mouth, but must travel down the guiding plane until the posterior retention is no longer effective (Fig 2-31). For this reason, the guiding planes created on the abutment teeth must be as long as possible in the all tooth-borne case.

Connectors

Major connector design for the mandibular Class III RPD remains basically the same as for the other classes. Again, whenever possible in the mandible, the lingual bar is selected over the lingual plate to reduce the amount of soft tissue coverage. As in the Class II, consideration must be given to the conversion of the casting to a distal extension base when the choice of a posterior terminal abutment is questionable.

Selecting a design for the maxillary connector that will provide adequate strength without bulk and give the patient maximum comfort is more of a challenge. The broad palatal strap design forms the basis of all maxillary major connectors. Modifications will depend on the number and position of the edentulous areas. Major connectors can be kept to a thickness of 0.5 mm if they are planned so that they cover a portion of the slope of the rugae area as well as the vault of the posterior palate; this forms a corrugation in the basic form, which increases the rigidity of the connector. Again, cantilevers from more posterior rests can be used to replace single anterior teeth and still leave the speaking area of the palate open.

Resin Retention

Since there is seldom any need to reline a Class III RPD, resin retention will be metal ridge coverage with retentive beads, loops, or posts and the occasional metal pontic. These metal pontics can be veneered or, in the posterior where they will not be visible, left in metal. The full metal pontic should not extend buccally as it would if it were being veneered. By keeping it lingual to the buccal line angle, its presence can be disguised.

Clasping

Clasping is limited to the posterior abutments of the Class III RPD whenever possible, because the potential for parallel guiding planes adjacent to the edentulous spaces is great and will eliminate the need for anterior clasping in all but those situations where the clinical crowns are so short that no adequate guiding planes can be created. As the crowns get shorter, the need to have parallel planes increases—a real challenge in subtractive mouth preparation. Guiding planes that are additive have the advantage of allowing machined milling to create "perfect" parallelism. The clasp of choice for the posterior will be the cast circumferential placed into a 0.010-inch undercut for the terminal third of the active clasp arm. The need for anterior clasping can best be determined after the casting has been fitted. Should retention appear inadequate at that time, one or more distal wire I-bars can be added to the framework into a 0.010-inch undercut.

Class IV RPD

The Class IV partial denture patient classification represents a group of patients for whom the advent of osseointegrated implants has greatly reduced the reliance on the removable partial denture. Most of these patients go through a stage of treatment in which a cast partial denture is essential, even though the final prosthesis may be implant supported and retained. The cost of a casting is insignificant when compared with the possible problems of long-term all-resin provisionals. For these patients, as well as those for whom no implant-supported or fixed prosthodontics is possible or affordable, the Class IV RPD represents a challenge both in design and construction. A special type of partial denture, using a rotational path of insertion/removal, has great potential in the Class IV maxillary situation and will be addressed later (see Chapter 9).

Abutment Selection

For the most part, the patient with an extensive anterior edentulous space will need the support of all the remaining teeth. Those with smaller edentulous areas will require at least the teeth adjacent to the edentulous area and the first molars. Again, the more

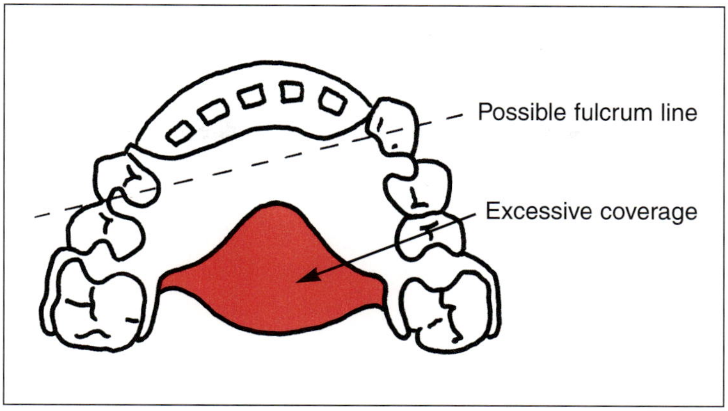

Fig 2-32 Extension in palate may rotate away from tissue in function.

teeth being replaced on the partial and the weaker the quality of the abutments, either periodontally or restoratively, the more teeth that must be involved as abutments. For the other classifications, the path of insertion/removal was planned to be in the long axis of the abutment teeth so as to load them vertically as much as possible and to reduce to the very minimum the amount of tooth structure lost to mouth preparation for guiding planes. For the Class IV situation, consideration must be given to the undercuts in the flange area because, if a full flange is desired, these soft tissue undercuts will have to draw with the posterior guiding planes. It is often impossible to make this alignment without crowning the abutment teeth. Another solution is to plan on a short flange only, one that extends just to the height of contour of the edentulous ridge when the path of insertion/removal favors the abutment teeth. Decisions on this dilemma are often based on the need for a full flange to restore lip support.

Connectors

Mandibular major connectors for this classification offer the same options as the other mandibular designs. They are more apt to be full lingual plates, since the necessary additional frictional retention can be obtained from the preparation of parallel guiding planes on the lingual surfaces of the remaining teeth. The continuous lingual plate gives the maximum contact with these surfaces.

Maxillary major connectors will often differ somewhat from those used for other classifications. Since the edentulous area is apt to be extensive, ie, greater than that which would normally be replaced with a fixed partial denture, rotational movements around an axis that will run between the most mesial rigid contact of the framework and the anterior abutment on each side can be expected. As rotation of the base toward the tissue takes place, any portion of the major connector that is posterior to this fulcrum will have a tendency to move away from the tissue (Fig 2-32). The farther posterior the casting extends, the greater the potential for breaking contact with the soft tissue. The space that may be opened up here can act as a food trap during mastication. To reduce this rotational opening, the posterior extension of the major connector should be limited and should never extend beyond the posterior clasping.

While it may appear that the open oval or anterior-posterior bar configuration is appropriate for the Class IV situation, the palatal extension of the anterior segment can still interfere with speech unless it is carefully blended with the contour of the anterior rugae area.

The rotational path Class IV option requires additional decisions on major connector design (see Chapter 9).

Resin Retention

Most Class IV cases will require raised mesh retention because the edentulous spans are apt to be extensive and therefore may need future relines to keep the partial stable. Since the external finishing line of the maxillary partial will lie in the speaking area, some consideration should be given to blending the junction of the metal and the resin in such a way as to eliminate a ridge in the area where speech is formed. This may require moving the finishing line posteriorly or bringing it almost to the denture teeth, depending on the palatal contour.

Clasping

A conventional Class IV partial will have its primary retention on the molar teeth (usually the first molars), one on each side. These clasps will often be cast circumferential, either coming from a modification space or as an embrasure clasp. In the maxillary arch, the anterior edentulous area often requires an additional clasp to offset the pull of gravity and sticky foods. When long parallel guiding planes are obtainable adjacent to the edentulous area, the casting may be retentive without the third clasp. Since the anterior clasp is likely to be visible and possibly unesthetic, the casting should be evaluated without the anterior clasp. When additional retention is required, the third clasp is added as a wire I-bar soldered to the casting.

The mandibular Class IV will not usually need a third clasp if guiding planes are well-planned and executed. If the guiding planes are inadequate, the same approach for the third clasp should be used.

This chapter has covered the basis of removable partial denture design. The keys to success are careful and exacting preparation of a healthy mouth and control of the tooth-frame relationship through attention to detail in the laboratory. The clinician who follows the principles established here will find design decisions reduced to a minimum. The anatomy of the mouth and the number and location of the missing teeth will greatly influence the decision, leaving personal preference as only a modifying factor. Prosthodontists do not, as a rule, wear removable partial dentures and so have no feeling for the patient's response to the addition of so much material in the mouth. Clinicians can, however, make a casting or two to fit their mouths and at least evaluate the placement and configuration of the major connector. Many of the ideas expressed here have come from just that experience.

3

Mouth Preparation

Mouth preparation, as described earlier, covers everything we do to prepare the mouth for the actual construction of the removable partial denture. Restorative procedures associated with the remaining teeth are obviously a responsibility of the primary clinician, but most other areas of mouth preparation fall under the management of specialists or general practitioners with expertise in the areas of periodontal therapy, endodontics, orthodontics, and oral and maxillofacial surgery.

For the most part, mouth preparation is looked upon as preparing a few rest seats, perhaps a surveyed crown or two, and then getting on with the final impression for the casting. Since mouth preparation is the foundation for all we plan to do later on, it is essential that a planning phase be developed. All possible changes required to bring the mouth to an optimum state of health must be identified, with the remaining dentition properly aligned and positioned, so that the resulting partial denture can be as ideal as is humanly possible. Mouth preparation for the state-of-the-art RPD requires diagnostic procedures that include, but are not limited to, the following:

- Survey of the diagnostic cast with selection of the path of insertion/removal.
- Reshaping of stone teeth to ideal contours for subtractive mouth preparation.
- Diagnostic waxing of any areas requiring additive mouth preparation.
- Diagnostic set-up of teeth to be replaced.
- Orthodontic set-up for teeth requiring minor tooth movement.
- Ridge mapping for gingival surgery and implants.
- Creation of a preparation guide (vacuum-formed) for surveyed crowns.
- Centric relation records, and mounting of diagnostic and opposing casts (where indicated).
- Impressions, jaw relation records, and esthetic set-up of opposing arch (if totally or partially edentulous).

Only when these extensive diagnostic procedures have been completed, the definitive treatment plan developed, a treatment plan letter for informed consent written and signed by the patient, and all consults finished, should the actual irreversible mouth preparation begin.

Surveying the Diagnostic Cast

When the diagnostic cast has been mounted in the survey table, the easiest way to begin the survey process is to stand over the cast and, using the parallax of the eyes, attempt to look down the long axes of the abutment teeth. The prime abutment(s), should they exist (as in Class I and II situations), will determine the path of insertion/removal for the partial since the guiding plane established on the distal surface of the prime abutment will be the key to the remaining mouth preparation. This position is found by tilting the cast in the sagittal plane. Once the anterior-posterior position has been determined, possible retentive areas can be equalized by tilting the cast in the frontal plane. Before tripoding the cast, all proximal surfaces that will have guiding planes and all potential retentive undercuts are verified using the analyzing rod in the surveyor. Minor adjustments to the tilt are then made and tripod marks placed on the cast. The tripod marks should be in such a position that they can all be seen at one time. Vertical markings on the sides of the land areas, while they do allow accurate repositioning, are much more difficult to use because they cannot all be seen at one glance. When the marks are widely spread out, one on the lingual of the anterior area and the other two on the lingual lateral surfaces of the retromolar pads or tuberosities, the cast can be easily repositioned by clinician and technician alike.

At this point the lead is placed in the surveyor and the entire height of contour of all teeth that will possibly be contacted by the partial is marked. Edentulous areas require the identification of their heights of contour as well. Without information on both hard and soft tissue undercuts, there is insufficient data on which to base the design and the mouth preparation that will be needed.

A reasoned design needs to be carefully drawn on the diagnostic cast before diagnostic mouth preparation can begin. It makes sense to use a color code that is familiar to your laboratory. Making a neat and precise drawing on a stone cast is not as easy as it would appear, and most diagnostic casts seen in the dental laboratory will have drawings that are childish at best. None of us has a natural talent for drawing in three planes. All our previous efforts in drawing have been done on the two dimensions of a piece of paper. To simulate the two-dimensional drawing with which we are familiar, the cast is braced against the clinician's stomach and rotated with one hand while the other hand draws. In this way the pencil stays in the comfortable two-plane position while the third plane is managed via the rotation of the cast. Just a little practice will allow even the "non-artist" to make a credible drawing. There is an added value to having a neatly constructed design drawing: technicians are much more likely to give their best effort when the materials submitted to them are of the highest quality. The well-drawn design on the diagnostic cast reinforces the level of quality desired in the final prosthesis.

Diagnostic Mouth Preparation

Perhaps the most important step in the construction of a removable partial denture is the preparation of the diagnostic cast. The process is broken down into subtractive mouth preparation, that is, the reduction of existing tooth contours to some predetermined ideal state, and additive mouth preparation, the diagnostic waxing of contours that must be altered with fixed appliances, be they crowns, bonded metal guiding planes or bonded composite rest seats.

Subtractive mouth preparation is done first, using the same instrumentation that will be used in the actual tooth recontouring. The armamentarium will include:

- Both tapered and nontapered diamond cylinders of medium/fine grit for the preparation of the guiding planes
- Round diamonds for occlusal rest preparation in either 8D, 10D, or 12D
- Inverted cone for cingulum preparation in 37 or 39 size

Using the actual clinical diamonds on the stone teeth does not harm the diamonds and offers the opportunity to practice the preparations. The stone teeth are to be prepared to ideal contour even though it may not be possible to do so in the mouth. Once the practice subtractive mouth preparation is completed, a decision on the clinical possibility of creating the same preparation on the natural tooth is made on a tooth-to-tooth basis. Obviously, there will be many instances when compromises will have to be made between the ideal and the possible. For some of these situations, the actual design may be changed, orthodontic minor tooth movement required, or additive mouth preparation undertaken to achieve the ideal situation.

The sequence of subtractive mouth preparation must always be guiding planes first, followed by rest seat preparation. Once the stone teeth have been prepared, the design is redrawn to its original state. Dimensions and depths of rest seat preparation should be ideal, once again, with possible compromises or changes in design coming after intraoral reevaluation.

Additive preparation follows with the diagnostic waxing of crowns and bonded contours. The surveyor blade is used to create "milled" guiding plane surfaces on the waxups, again, to ideal contours. When full crowns are desired for the abutment teeth in Class III and IV partials, the proximal guiding planes will be extended as far as possible so that maximum frictional retention can be obtained (Fig 3-1). The contours of bonded restorations are waxed directly on the diagnostic cast. The design of the base of bonded castings will be identical to those of the bonded fixed partial denture (Maryland bridge or Rochette style). The contours of bonded composite restorations, usually cingulum rest seats for mandibular canines and guiding planes, are also waxed to ideal contours. Retentive areas for clasps are to be brought as close as possible to the gingiva, leaving a minimum of 1 mm of space between the proposed clasp arm and the soft tissue, a task easily accomplished in the waxing of a crown but not always possible in natural tooth structure or bonded metal or composite. Since the crown gives us the potential for creating the ideal abutment contour, thought must be given to the timing of the undercut.

The relationship of the height of contour to the desired undercut depth determines

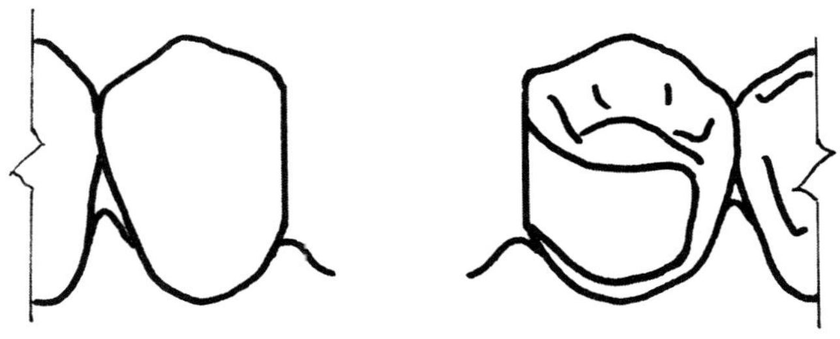

Fig 3-1 Guiding planes fully extended.

the quality of retention that will occur when the retentive clasp dislodges from the tooth. If there is some distance (a gradual transition) between the height of contour and the desired undercut (0.01 to 0.015 inch), then the resulting retention will be apt to be weaker but last for a longer time as the clasp moves toward the height of contour. If the undercut is steep (that is, with little distance between the 0.01-inch point and the height of contour), then the initial retention is apt to be greater, but it will not last as long (Fig 3-2). The gradual undercut is best suited for a distal extension situation (Class I) in the mandibular arch. This will allow a certain amount of stress relief in the clasp-tooth relationship. The steeper undercut area is more apt to be used in a tooth-borne situation in the maxilla where the patient will appreciate maximum retention against the force of gravity. These decisions on contour are made at this time so that a diagnostic record of the ideal contour of the abutment teeth will be available throughout the treatment phase and not have to be redesigned at each subsequent step in treatment.

The final step in the diagnostic preparation of the mouth is to position the replacement denture teeth. The denture teeth will have to be ordered from the dental manufacturer at some time during treatment, so the earlier, the better. The criteria for shade selection will be the same no matter when the selection is made. The mold can best be determined from an analysis of the diagnostic cast as soon as it is recovered. The definitive denture teeth can therefore be readily available to the clinician at the time of diagnostic mouth preparation. An alternative is to use teeth from a mold guide for diagnostic procedures and bring in the actual denture teeth later on; however, if some tooth modification is necessary, the continued recontouring of the mold guide teeth may be unacceptable.

A quick wax procedure for isolated missing teeth can be accomplished by selecting a tooth from the mold guide and impressing it in alginate. When the alginate is set, the denture tooth is removed and molten wax poured in the mold. The wax tooth is modified to fit the edentulous area on the cast and waxed to place.

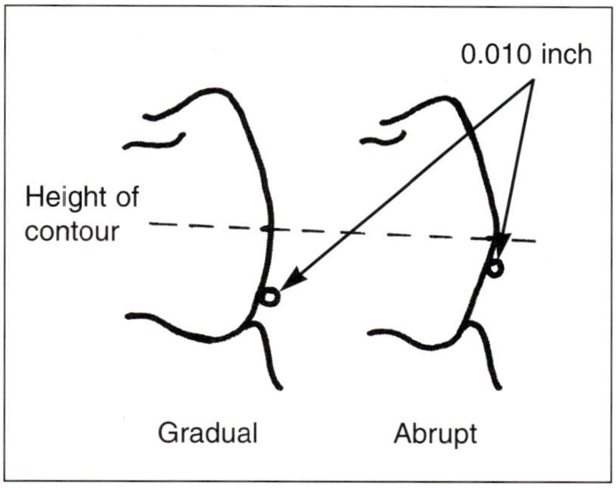

Fig 3-2 Quality and quantity of retention.

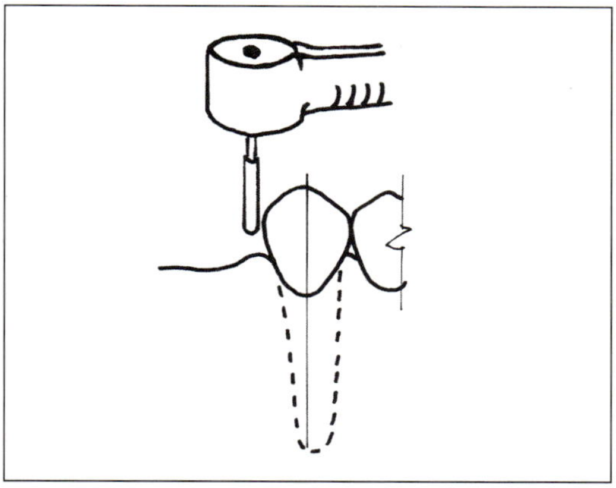

Fig 3-3 The long axis of a prime abutment is used to establish the first guiding plane.

With the denture teeth in position, the diagnostic procedure is complete and the patient can be shown the recontoured cast as a means of describing the treatment plan (another reason for a quality drawing and a clean and neat cast).

Clinical Mouth Preparation

Subtractive Mouth Preparation

The actual subtractive mouth preparation is begun using the diagnostic ideal mouth preparation from the cast as a template. Preparing parallel guiding planes in the mouth can only be accomplished with practice. Clinicians trained in the era of multiple pinledge restorations will recall the paralleling devices that were attached to teeth not involved in the restoration so that the contra-angle handpiece could be kept in the same plane throughout the preparations. That type of device is not usable for the preparation of guiding planes, since teeth on both sides of the arch are involved. The best guide available to the clinician is the reference of the long axis of the prime abutment and the angle of the predetermined guiding plane to that long axis (Fig 3-3). If no prime abutment exists, the tooth that offers the clinician the greatest visibility and accessibility is chosen to act as the indicator for the first guiding plane. After the first pass with the diamond cylinder, the resulting guiding plane is visually evaluated against the prepared surface of the stone cast and, if the planes appear to be identical, further refinement of the proximal surface is carried out. From that point on, the clinician refers back to the original guiding plane to set the angle of the diamond cylinder before moving on to the other abutments. After all the guiding planes have been prepared, an alginate impression is made and poured in fast-set plaster to serve as a check cast. This cast, when recovered, is placed on the surveyor, and the guiding planes are evaluated for parallelism. Any discrepancies are adjusted on the cast and then corrected in the mouth.

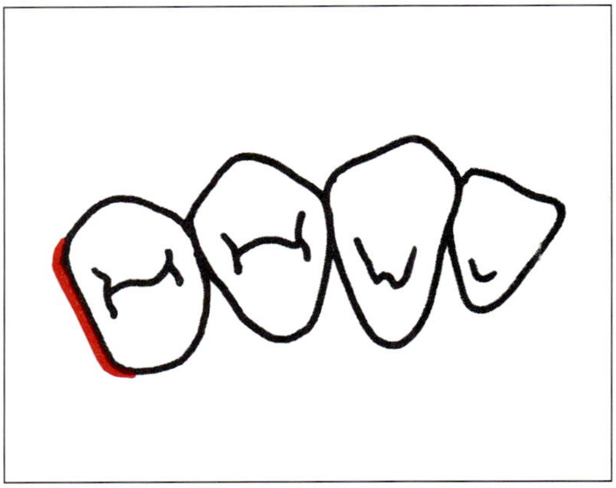

Fig 3-4 Buccal and lingual extension of guiding plane.

Remember, guiding planes for Class II, III, and IV should be as long as possible vertically without compromising the enamel. In some situations in the older mouth, the guiding planes can be taken into dentin. By preparing the teeth without anesthesia, the patient can indicate when the tooth becomes sensitive and the extent of the guiding plane can be reevaluated. The buccolingual dimension of the guiding plane in these three situations should extend just around the line angle in most cases. This slight extension, the turning of the "corner," will greatly enhance reciprocation and provide the bracing component that used to be dependent on the bracing clasp arm (Fig 3-4). The only exception to the buccal extension of this plane would be on the mesial proximal surface of a tooth in the anterior portion of the mouth, where the guide plate of the partial could be seen and be unesthetic (most likely in the Class IV).

For the Class I RPD, the clinician will have to choose between the shorter guiding plane with the stress relief "built in" and the longer guiding plane that will require functional adaptation of the guide plate on the casting for the same amount of stress relief. Both of these designs have been proven to be effective in allowing some level of stress relief. The shorter guiding plane, with its guide plate touching the tooth only at the gingival extension of the plane, requires a more precise level of laboratory support; this is unfortunate because it would appear to offer control with the least amount of adjusting at the chair. When the laboratory support is less than ideal, the longer guiding plane and plate will be more apt to provide contact of these surfaces. The Class IV situation has often been described as a Class I in reverse and, if stress relief is indicated (when the remaining abutment teeth are less than ideal supports), the decision as to the prime guiding planes on the mesial of the most anterior teeth will have to be made on the same basis as for the Class I. However, when a rotational path RPD is planned, the proximal undercut must be maintained, thus eliminating the guiding plane adjacent to the edentulous area.

Once the guiding planes have been prepared and verified, the occlusal rest seats are prepared. The tendency has always been to make the rest seats too small and to leave them with sharp angles or with undercuts to the path of insertion/removal (especially in the case of the isolated mandibular molar, where the rest may draw by itself, usually to the mesiolingual, but will not draw with the other guiding planes, resulting in a casting that will not fully seat). The rest seats are to be one third the buccolingual dimension of the tooth. The rest seat must be deep enough to allow for 1.2 mm of metal in the rest. A round diamond with the same diameter as the desired rest seat should be selected. The occlusal rest has historically been presented as needing to be "spoon shaped," meaning that the seat is deeper in the center of the

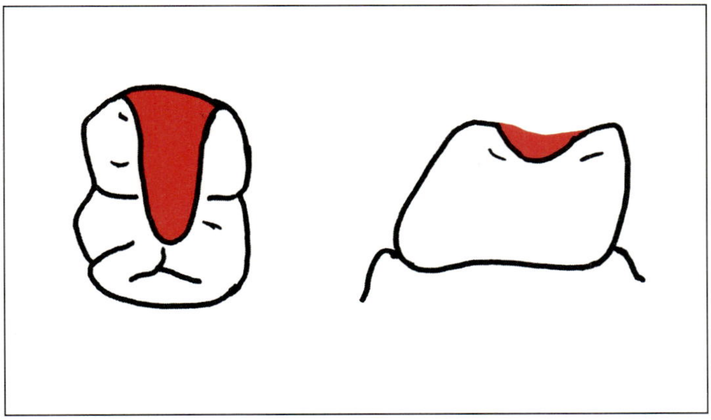

Fig 3-5 Ideal rest seat dimensions for the isolated mandibular molar.

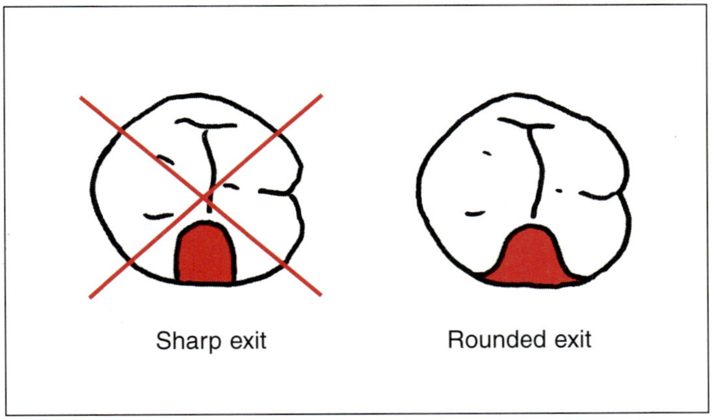

Fig 3-6 Proper rest seat contour at the marginal ridge.

tooth than it is at the marginal ridge. Unfortunately, this results in a marginal ridge without adequate space for metal and in a casting that will eventually break right at the marginal rest—a difficult repair situation. The rest seat on any isolated tooth, and especially on a single mandibular molar, should extend at least to the center of the occlusal surface so that the rest can direct the occlusal forces down the long axis of the abutment (Fig 3-5).

After the bulk of the occlusal rest seat has been prepared, attention must be paid to the junction of the guiding plane and the rest seat. The sharp line that results from the intersection of the two surface reductions must be rounded (Fig 3-6). To leave this sharp angle is to risk a casting that will not fully seat, since the thin, sharp edge is unlikely to stand up in the refractory. If even a slight defect in this area is created during the formation of the refractory cast or in the waxing of the framework, a positive bleb will result. Clinical studies of the fit of partial denture castings indicate that the marginal ridge area is where the greatest amount of contact can be expected.

When placing occlusal rest seats in amalgam restorations, there is always the possibility of weakening the alloy in the depth of the rest or along the vertical walls. Should the amalgam appear to be

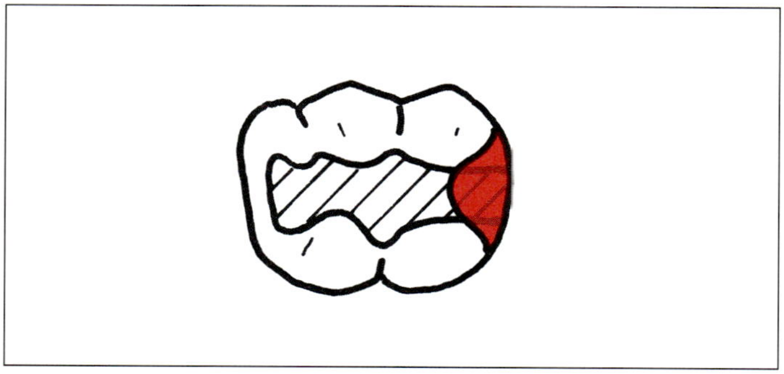

Fig 3-7 Rest preparation extended beyond alloy margin.

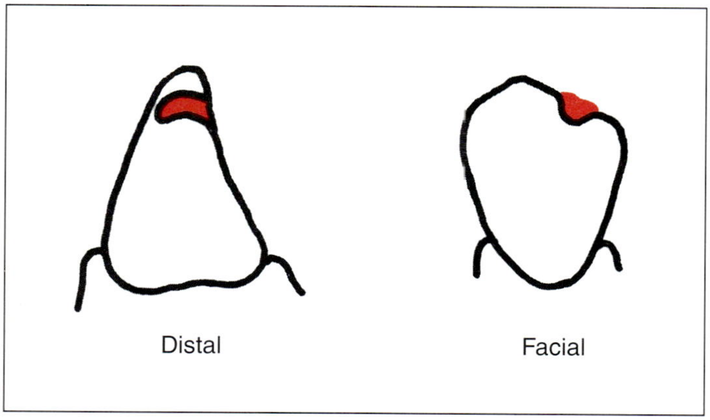

Fig 3-8 Incisal rest is used primarily on distal aspect of mandibular canines.

compromised, it must be redone with greater extensions. An alternative would be to consider a casting. If there is no opposing occlusion or if the occlusion is with a denture tooth, the rest preparation can be extended beyond the margins of the old alloy and the depth of the preparation can be reduced (Fig 3-7). The demands of the thickness of the rest remain, but this space can be developed, at least in part, at the expense of the opposing denture tooth. Occlusal rest preparations in existing crowns are another area of concern, since there is no way of evaluating the thickness of the occlusal metal or metal-porcelain. The patient must be informed that if a perforation occurs during mouth preparation, the crown must be remade. Sometimes a design change can eliminate the need to prepare a certain tooth. Often, though, the treatment plan will have to include the new crown as a distinct possibility.

Incisal rest seats are prepared in the same manner as for the occlusal rest. The diamond of choice is the tapered cylinder rather than the round bur since the ideal incisal rest is one that is rounded both mesiodistally and buccolingually, without undercuts, of course, to the path of insertion/removal. Here again, the junction of the seat with the guiding plane must be rounded (Fig 3-8).

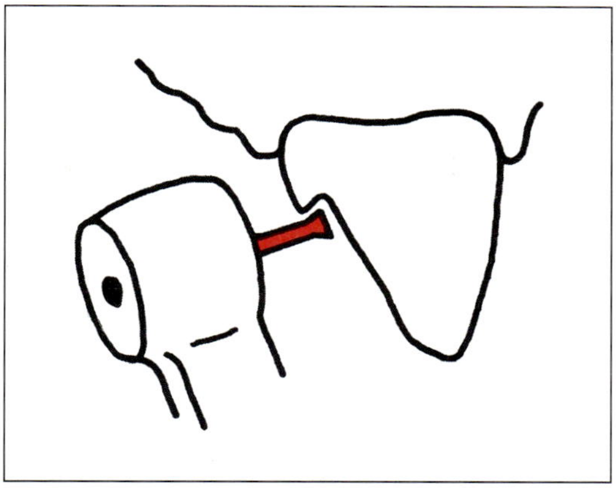

Fig 3-9 Proper angulation of inverted cone diamond stone for cingulum rest on maxillary canine.

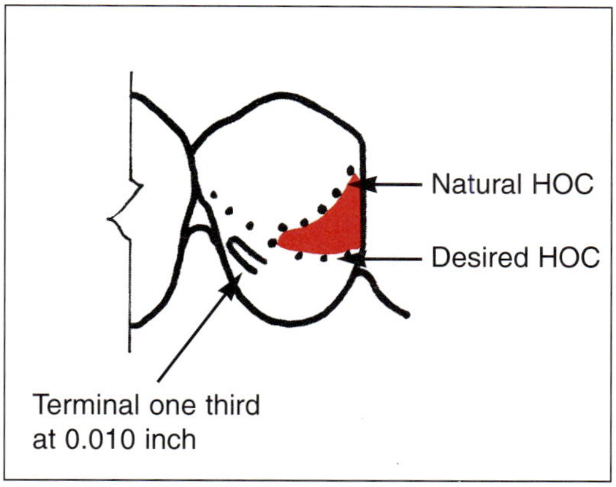

Fig 3-10 Required reduction for the proximal two thirds of a retentive clasp arm. HOC = Height of contour.

Cingulum rests, limited to maxillary canines for the most part, are prepared with a diamond inverted cone (Fig 3-9). The size of the cone is determined by the bulk of enamel in the cingulum. The greater the amount of enamel, the larger the rest seat can be. It is also possible to augment the rest seat with bonded composite to create a rest with a floor of 1.5 mm. The reason a diamond is chosen over a carbide inverted cone is that the diamond leaves a more rounded internal angle. If this area is sharp, the same problems can arise as with the marginal ridge. The shape of the rest seat as seen from the lingual is one of an inverted "V," which follows the natural shape of the cingulum and requires the minimum reduction of tooth structure.

Cingulum rest seats on maxillary anteriors are often required and, if sufficient enamel exists below the contact of the mandibular incisors, they are prepared with the same inverted cone as the canine, the only difference being the shape of the rest. It is more apt to be straight or semilunar, as it follows the natural contour of the lingual gingival surface. These rest seats often require augmentation.

Additional reduction is often required on the buccal and lingual surfaces of posterior teeth to drop the height of contour closer to the gingiva (especially on lingually inclined mandibular posteriors). The approach arms of minor connectors will need a minor guiding plane gingival to the marginal ridge for additional frictional retention. When circumferential clasp arms are planned, the proximal two thirds must lie at or slightly above the height of contour. Since the tooth at the line angle normally has the contour rising to the marginal ridge, reduction in this area is required to bring the proximal portion toward the gingiva and out of possible occlusal interference (Fig 3-10). These contours are best reduced with a nontapered cylinder. As guiding planes enter the lingual embrasures on their way to the supplementary rests, it may be necessary to change to a finely tapered, diamond cylinder just to get into the constricted space. The guiding planes can still be kept

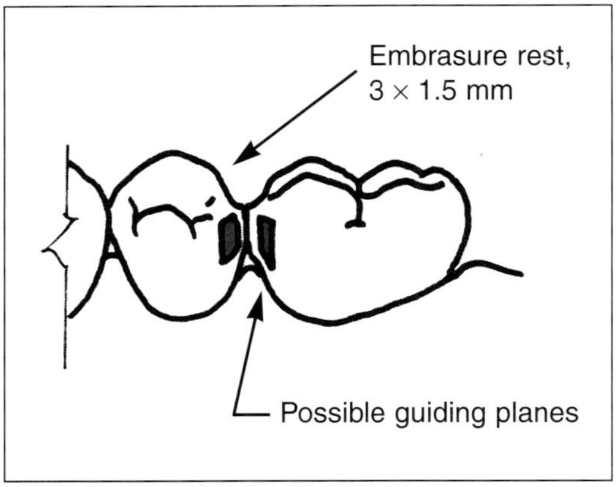

Fig 3-11 Lingual mouth preparation for embrasure clasp.

parallel to the proposed path of insertion by slightly tilting the handpiece so that the tapered cylinder cuts at 90 degrees (parallel to other guiding planes).

Embrasure clasps require preparation in addition to the rest seat. Depending upon the contact area of the marginal ridges and the opposing occlusion, an access must be established for the clasp arm to both enter and exit the rest area. The exit to the buccal surface is usually the most critical. In either case, a minimum of 1.5 mm of space, both vertically and horizontally, must be created. A tapered diamond cylinder is used to create the space, cutting at 1.5 mm on the cylinder for automatic control of the dimension. The lingual approach to the marginal ridge offers the possibility of a minor guiding plane that should always be used, since the embrasure clasp assembly offers no other possibility of a guiding plane (Fig 3-11). The rest seat area is to be shared between the two adjacent teeth to conserve tooth structure and still have adequate space for the rest. Under no circumstance should the contact actually be broken. If it is broken by mistake, a restoration will have to be placed on one of the contacting teeth to restore contact. When a restricted space is left for the embrasure clasp, fracture of the retentive clasp arm can be expected. The plastic pattern used to wax the clasp has a cross-sectional measurement of approximately 1.5 mm; should any reduction be necessary on the occlusal portion of the clasp, an area of stress concentration will occur and fracture can be expected after repeated flexure. Repair of a broken clasp arm in the embrasure area is difficult and cannot be depended on.

Guiding planes are usually not prepared on anterior teeth because reshaping of the proximal surfaces alters the shape of the tooth to the point where esthetics is compromised. Occasionally, a minor guiding plane can be created on lingual surfaces where gingival recession or crown lengthening leaves the full anatomic crown exposed.

When inadequate space is available for an anterior replacement, the adjacent teeth may be recontoured to equalize the pontic space with the adjacent teeth. When the space is so constricted that an esthetic result is not attainable, orthodontics or a fixed partial denture replacement may be the only options.

At the completion of the subtractive mouth preparation, the surfaces that have been recontoured must be finished and polished. Since these prepared surfaces should be the only areas where contact between the tooth and the frame takes place, there are significant advantages to polishing with either a fine diamond or fine white stone followed by rubber points and disks. The chances of alginate sticking and tears are reduced. Since the refractory material required for stellate alloys is large grained, the exact duplication of irregular surfaces is not possible. The resultant casting will be apt to have an internal surface that is naturally rough, so every effort should be made to reduce this surface roughness.

Additive Mouth Preparation

Before any preparation is undertaken for additive contours, the subtractive component of the mouth preparation must be complete to include final polish. It is obviously easier to create a casting in harmony with the contours already established on the teeth than to make the casting first and try to create guiding planes on the teeth to match those on the casting.

Additive mouth preparation can be broken down into three different approaches to obtaining ideal contour: bonded metal contours, composite contours, and more traditional surveyed crowns and pontics. The actual contours established using these modalities are the same, only the means of connecting them to the abutment teeth differ. Both bonded metal contours and crowns require mouth preparation of enamel surfaces as a part of their construction. All bonded restorations require the presence of sound tooth structure, preferably enamel, to which to bond.

Bonded Metal Contours

Rest seat areas, guiding planes, and attachments all lend themselves to bonding to enamel. They offer a high level of predictability but are technique sensitive. The more attention to detail during the preparation of the enamel, the greater the long-term success.

The cingulum rest seat, to be placed on the lingual slope of a mandibular canine, is the most commonly used bonded contour. The mouth preparation for this restoration is limited to a horizontal notch cut in the enamel in the gingival third of the lingual slope. This miniature cingulum rest serves as a vertical stop when seating the casting at cementation and as a positioning device to relate the restoration in its proper position. Since the enamel on the lingual of the mandibular canine is thin, this groove will not be more than 0.5 mm in depth to be certain to stay in enamel. Although not really necessary, one can reduce 0.2 mm of enamel overall and leave a finishing line so that the resultant casting, which will be approximately 0.4 mm thick, will have a smoother interface with the surrounding tooth structure.

When guiding planes are incorporated on the casting, microgroove preparations, as recommended by Schärer and Marinello, are placed in the enamel using the smallest-diameter slightly tapered carbide bur (Fig 3-12). These grooves offer lateral resistance to dislodgment and have been shown to greatly increase the successful bond between casting and tooth. (Precision attachment castings are discussed in Chapter 10.)

Final impressions for bonded castings are made in either silicone or polyether, since they are poured in the refractory material that is compatible with the alloy to be used. These refractory materials do not, as a rule, set against alginate. The impression need not be full arch but must contain the other prepared abutments so that any guiding plane area on the casting can be made parallel with the existing guiding planes. If the base of the casting extends to the gingiva, a retraction cord should be placed to assure accuracy in that area.

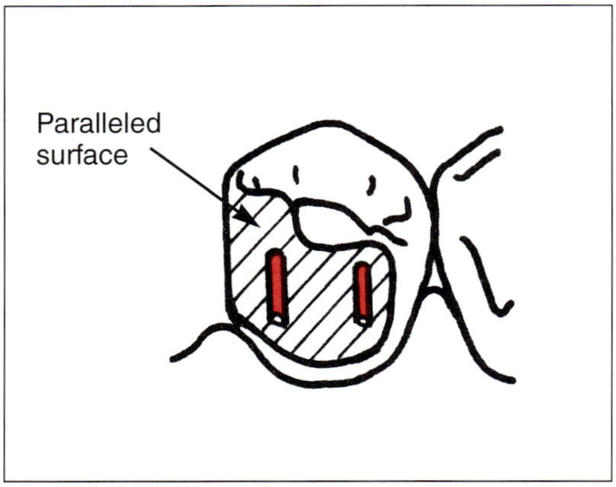

Fig 3-12 Microgroove preparation for bonded castings.

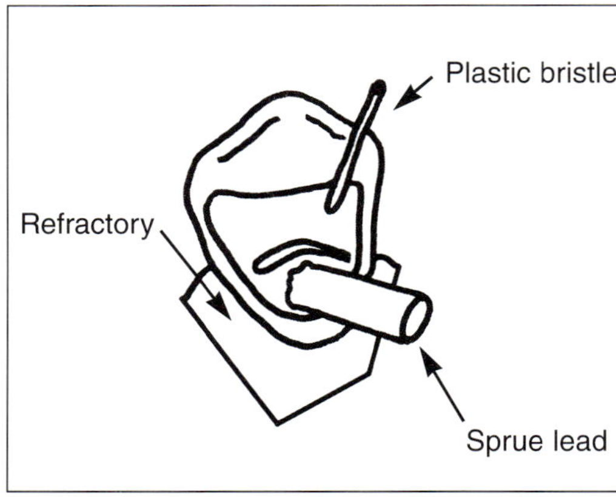

Fig 3-13 Sprued wax pattern on sectioned refractory cast.

The borders of the casting are outlined, and a small piece of sheet wax, available from Kerr Laboratory Products Division at 0.5 mm thickness, is adapted to the outline and waxed to place by adding a small amount of very hot wax all around the border. The contours of the restoration are added to this wax base. For a cingulum rest, the base must have a width of 1.2 mm with a rounded internal angle. The rest must form an acute angle to the path of insertion/removal so that it will be "positive" rest. Decisions on the contour and extent of any guiding planes must be made relative to the classification of the edentulous situation and the established contours of the other abutment teeth.

The wax-up is sprued with a round wax sprue attached to the lingual surface of the cingulum. As a final addition, a plastic bristle from a toothbrush is attached near the incisal or occlusal margin to act as a holding device for the casting during finishing and cementation (Fig 3-13). Since the pattern is waxed against a refractory cast, no attempt is made to remove the pattern. The refractory cast is cut with a die saw so that only a minimum of stone is present. The sprue is then attached to the base of a casting ring and the second stage of the investment is poured. The material of choice for the bonded casting is some form of Ni-Cr alloy (Rexillium or similar alloy).

The completed casting is finished and polished and, if it has a guiding plane, returned to a master cast for final milling using a milling machine. It is then prepared for either microretention through an etching process (as for a Maryland bridge) or for macroretention using countersunk perforations (Rochette). Either electrochemical or acid preparation of the internal surface is acceptable to etch the metal. Care must be taken not to contaminate the etched surface once the etching is complete. The holding device, cast from the plastic bristle, is used to hold the casting during cementation with a chemically cured composite. Light-cured composites can be used with the perforated design. Once the resin is cured under rubber dam, the holding device is cut from the casting and that area is stoned and rubber-wheeled to finish the restoration.

Bonded Resin Contours

Rest seats and guiding contours can also be established in composite alone. While it may appear that a restoration formed in composite would be likely to fracture when stressed repeatedly, experience of over 15 years has shown this not to be the case. When the abutment tooth has been properly managed, under rubber dam, and the composite placed according to the manufacturer's directions, this becomes a viable and less expensive alternative to the bonded cast contour.

The rest and/or guiding plane can be prepared in a bulk of bonded composite, as if it were enamel, or a template can be formed from the diagnostic wax-up to shape the composite as it is being bonded to the tooth. To create a working template, the diagnostic wax-up is duplicated in dental stone using alginate or reversible hydrocolloid. On the resulting cast, a vacuum-formed clear-plastic template is adapted and trimmed to contact the abutment tooth, as well as adjacent teeth on at least one side, to allow precise positioning during composite placement. A stone core is poured against the outer surface of the template to be used to force the template to place once it has been filled with composite.

After placement of the rubber dam, the tooth is etched and prepared according to the directions for the specific light-cured composite being used. The template is filled with composite to approximate the amount required to create the restoration and forced to place using the stone core (Fig 3-14). Once the template is fully seated, the core is removed and the composite cured using an intraoral light source through the template. The template is simply peeled away when the curing cycle is complete. Then the excess composite is removed, and the borders are finished and polished. Use of the template results in a superior finish because the bulk of the restoration will not need to be touched after curing. For a single simple cingulum rest seat, however, shaping a bulk of previously bonded composite is the most practical way to create the desired form.

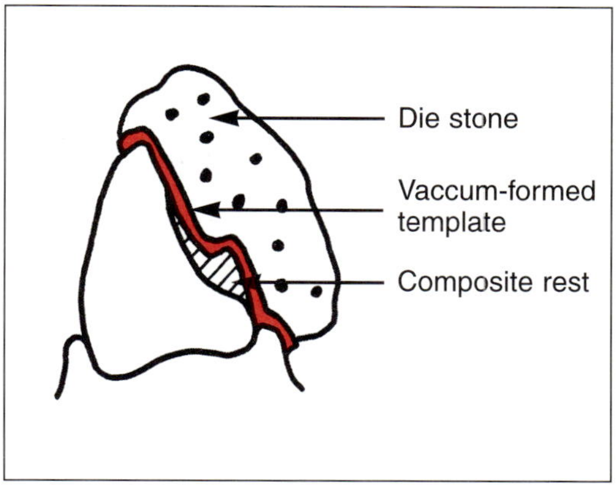

Fig 3-14 Template for composite cingulum rest.

When the composite used for these restorations is a microfill, the potential for wear is reduced. Unfortunately, all composites are somewhat brittle; therefore, when the abutment tooth is mobile, the bonded metal restoration is chosen be-

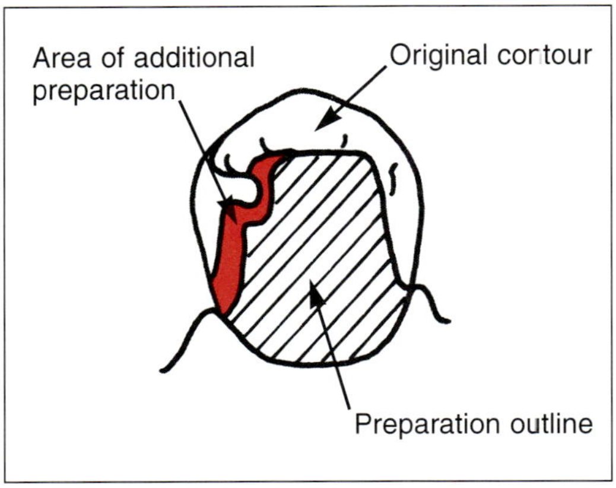

Fig 3-15 Subtractive mouth preparation before crown preparation.

cause the bulk of the all-composite restoration is more likely to fracture when the tooth is loaded during incision. The rest will be held by the partial denture while the tooth will be apt to move in the direction of the force applied, with the result of increased fracture caused by a shear of the bulk of the composite through the rest seat itself.

Both of these bonded options offer a relatively noninvasive approach to ideal mouth preparation with excellent reports of longevity for low cost. As previously stated, they require ample enamel for quality bonding.

Surveyed Crowns

The third and final form of additive mouth preparation is with the surveyed crown. This descriptive term has long been applied to any crown or pontic specially contoured and placed in conjunction with an abutment for a removable partial denture. Unfortunately, the crown, as obtained from the dental laboratory, is likely not to have the desired form as far as the partial denture is concerned, even though it may be ideal as a single-tooth restoration. The technician(s) who constructs the crown most likely will not have had partial denture experience and so will favor the contours of the natural crown. The modifications required by the ideal abutment may not be a part of that technician's training and, since the partial denture casting may well be constructed in a different laboratory, it will be the clinician's duty to control the contour of the crown.

Before beginning the mouth preparation phase of crown construction, the clinician must have gone through the diagnostic process of developing the ideal contour for the abutment tooth in question. The clinician must then prepare the tooth as if no crown were to be constructed: cut a guiding plane, prepare the rest seat, and make all other modifications of contour. Only then can the actual crown preparation begin. The initial subtractive mouth preparation will ensure that there has been adequate tooth reduction to allow the formation of the ideal contours in the final crown without compromising the restorative materials (Fig 3-15).

As a general rule, for veneered crowns, a disappearing margin or a metal collar should be used rather than a porcelain butt margin, since additional forces will be placed on the crown by the partial denture. Again, it is essential that all aspects of ideal soft tissue management be employed for the surveyed crown. Margin placement at or above the gingival margin, respect for the biologic width, and careful manipulation of retraction cord must be a part of the treatment.

The final impression for the crown will need to include more of the mouth than would the usual single-tooth impression. The entire denture-bearing space must be available on the master cast. This will insure that the plane of occlusion can be established independent of the maxillary teeth in complete denture (CD)/RPD situations by using the junction of the middle and distal third of the retromolar pad as the posterior determinate of the plane of occlusion, the anterior determinate being an anterior tooth that has not been prepared for a crown. The full cast will also allow the creation of a stable record base for jaw relation records should that be required. For any situation requiring multiple crowns, a patient-approved set-up of the CD/RPD is essential so that the plane of occlusion, as well as the relative position of the opposing denture teeth, has been definitively established. Obviously, all other abutment teeth must also be present on the master cast so that the additive mouth preparation can be in harmony with the previously completed subtractive preparation.

The only restriction on the dimensions and contour of the master cast is that it must fit into the survey table. Often this demand creates a problem when the distance of the base of the cast to the mounting ring is great, making the use of the dental surveyor and possibly the milling machine difficult if not impossible. Some modification of standard techniques is generally required, especially if the final impression is sent to the dental laboratory rather than being poured in clinic.

There is a distinct advantage, however, to pouring the cast, trimming the die(s), and mounting this type of case in the dental office: it allows the repositioning of the master cast for final determination of the path of insertion/removal and the placement of the three tripod marks on the cast. To expect the dental laboratory to complete all these steps and not lose control of the case requires a high level of experience and excellent and long-term communication between clinician and technician.

Until such time that a specific dental technician has been suitably trained and has demonstrated compliance with the requirements of a specific clinician, the "surveyed" crown is to be waxed to full contour and returned to the clinician for the actual shaping of all areas of crown–partial denture contact.

Since the ideal contours of the surveyed crown have been established in the diagnostic waxing phase of treatment planning, it should be a simple matter to copy the contours. Because of the critical nature of the "surveyed" surfaces in the long-term success of the treatment, it is essential to review the modifications to the full contour wax-up usually required to create the ideal crown. The first step is to reposition the master cast in the dental surveyor and reestablish the tilt of the cast to the original path of insertion/removal. It is to this path that we must evaluate the contours of the crown as returned from the laboratory. Dusting the wax with zinc stearate (or baby powder) will allow the analyzing rod of the dental surveyor to create an easily seen height of contour.

Using the blade that is normally a part of the components available for the surveyor or a wax milling bur in a dental milling device, the guiding planes are established parallel to any previously prepared planes in the enamel of the noncrowned teeth. Guiding planes can be cut as flat planes with or without a gingival ledge. The advantage of using the gingival ledge is that it

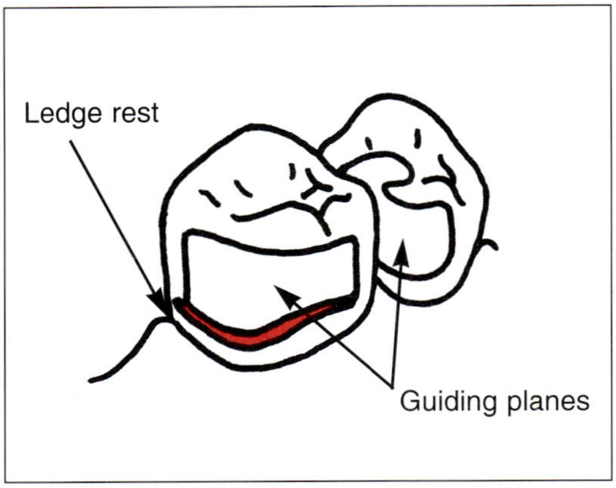

Fig 3-16 Guiding plane extensions.

functions as a rest and eliminates the need for an occlusal rest preparation. This is of particular value when esthetic demands require full porcelain occlusals. The guiding plane is not restricted to the proximal surface. In fact, the greater the extension of the guiding plane onto the lingual or buccal surface for reciprocation, the greater the frictional retention possibilities (Fig 3-16).

Only after all guiding plane surfaces have been contoured can we proceed to the placement of rest seats and retentive contours. It is essential that the junction of the guiding plane and rest is rounded and that sufficient wax has been removed to allow a minimum of 1.2 mm for any clasp/rest assembly. Rest preparations in crowns should be one third the occlusal table, which will often make them larger than they would be if cut into enamel. The larger and smoother the rest preparation, the greater chance that the partial denture will be in solid contact with it. One of the problems we face with every crown that will have a conventional clasp arm or arms is the determination of just where the height of contour is to be located in the wax-up. It is most desirable that any circumferential clasp lie as low on the tooth as is possible, both for esthetics and to maximize the retentive nature of the clasp arm. Since the die stone that represents the gingival marginal tissues has been removed from the die, an untrimmed second pour of the master impression is needed so that either clinician or technician can know the relation of the margin of the crown to the gingiva. We would like to place the inferior border of any circumferential clasp a full millimeter above the marginal tissue. The average cast clasp arm measures 1.5 mm occlusogingivally, so that the height of contour must be at least 2.5 mm above the tissue. Since we have the opportunity to make the crown contour truly ideal, a clinical, not laboratory, decision must be made as to the relation of the survey line to the final position of the clasp when the partial is fully seated. The greater the distance of the height of contour from the final clasp position, the longer lasting the retentive effect of the clasp will be. The flexing of the clasp will be more gradual, both on insertion and removal, but the initial retention will be reduced. It would seem then, that for all tooth-borne partials the height of contour should be close to the final position, perhaps 3 to 3.5 mm from the marginal tissue. This position will give a retentive force that is shorter acting but of greater initial value. For those situations where some level of stress relief is desired, it makes more sense to raise the height of contour to 4 to 4.5 mm from where the marginal tissue is known to be (Fig 3-17).

In addition to the creation or verification of the height of contour, the clinician must also determine the margin of the cutback for porcelain application. It is essential that a margin of metal exist beyond any extension of the partial framework so that guide plates, rests, and minor connectors contact

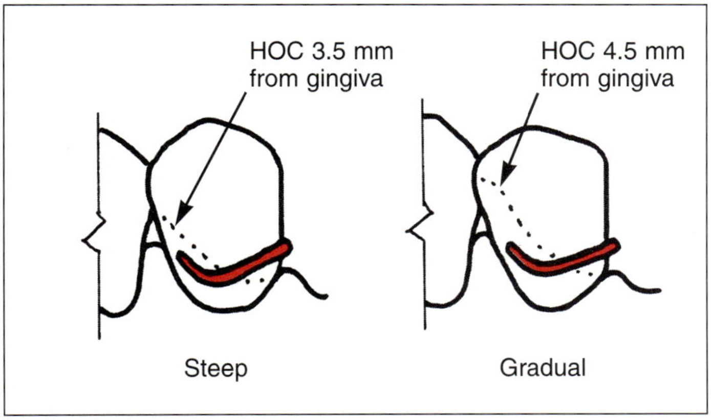

Fig 3-17 Options for retentive areas. HOC = Height of contour.

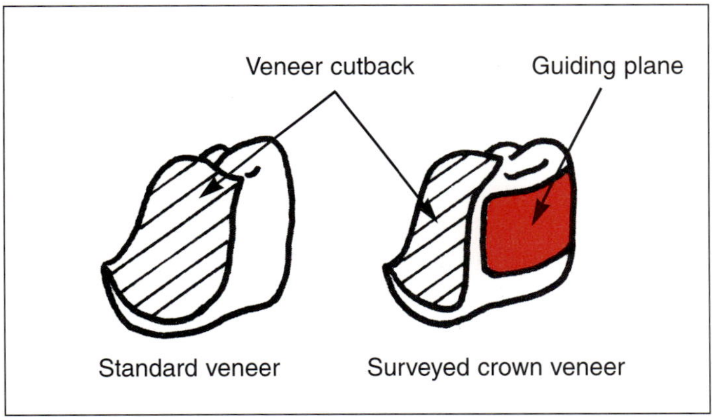

Fig 3-18 Options for cutback.

only the metal of the crown, not the porcelain. This margin need only be 0.5 mm. The resulting margin of the cutback will not be where it would be placed on a standard metal-ceramic restoration, so the technician needs to know exactly where to start the removal of wax. The clinician must outline the margin with an explorer so that there is no misunderstanding (Fig 3-18). Since the cutback will be a uniform reduction of the wax, allowing a uniform thickness of porcelain, it is essential that the wax crown has the exact contour desired in the final surveyed crown.

Even if the original contour was ideal and the cutback properly done, the application of the porcelain veneering, which must be done to excess because of the shrinkage factor, offers another opportunity to alter the height of contour and potentially render the crown unusable. For that reason it is advisable for the clinician to evaluate the crown after the porcelain is contoured at the bisque bake stage. Minor corrections of contour can easily be made by adding additional porcelain before final stain and glaze. The porcelain must be very smooth from the height of contour down to the final position of the clasp. If it is not, a dark line often becomes visible as the porcelain wears the metal of the clasp through repeated insertions and removals. Obviously, once the clinician and technician really understand each other, the technician can simply create an exact copy of the diagnostic wax-up.

The clinician has two options relative to combining these crowns and the partial denture framework. The crowns can either be cemented permanently before the final impression for the framework or they can be picked up in the final impression (which must then be made in a firm-setting elastomer-like Impregum). Resin dies must be constructed and be in the impression when it is poured so that they will be present on the master cast. It is impractical to include the single surveyed crown on the master cast, but for those situations where there are multiple surveyed crowns and bridges, with precise milling of their guiding surfaces, it is essential that the crowns be present on the master cast. The master cast will serve as the milling cast so that a stable base is available on which the final milling of the guiding planes is completed. The accuracy of the refractory cast is increased because the actual crowns, not stone replicas, were available for duplication. The final fit of the partial framework to the milled surfaces should therefore be enhanced. These special impression procedures are essential to the use of fixed restorations with precision attachments and will be discussed further in Chapter 10.

Mouth preparation, in the largest sense, when well-planned and executed, will simplify the actual construction of the advanced partial denture and ensure its long-term success. It is unfortunate that the great majority of removable partial dentures are made with little or limited regard to this crucial component of care. Remember, it is essential to establish all aspects of the mouth preparation on the diagnostic cast before any attempt is made to go to the mouth.

4

Final Impressions and Master Casts

Final impressions for removable partial denture frameworks are made in irreversible hydrocolloid in either modified stock trays or custom trays. Alginate is preferred over silicone or polyether materials because it will tear rather than distort. Remember, the silicone-type impression materials were designed for the impression of prepared teeth, where a minimum of undercuts will be found. The removable partial denture impression will often include unprepared teeth that may be severely tipped or rotated, leaving large undercuts that could well distort by tearing the impression material from the tray and may never be noticed until the casting does not fit the mouth. Since the contact surfaces between RPD and teeth are to be smooth, rounded, and well-polished, there is no need to reproduce minute detail as with the fixed prosthodontic impression materials. To use this tear phenomenon, the clinician must carefully evaluate the final impression under good light. As described in Chapter 1, in the section on preliminary impressions, the final impression should be relatively easy because the majority of potential problems were identified during those first impressions. Using the diagnostic cast, the adaptation of the stock tray can be evaluated; if the mandatory 0.25 inch is not available, a custom tray is made with adequate relief to assure the 0.25 inch of alginate. All custom alginate trays must have multiple retentive holes placed in them using a no. 8 or no. 10 round bur. These retentive holes combined with alginate adhesive will assure the retention of the impression material. It is obviously more important in the final than the preliminary impression to mix the alginate properly, place it into critical areas, and allow the complete set of the material. If the preliminary impression is taken seriously, however, there will be no difference in the techniques employed to obtain an accurate master cast.

The final impression is to be poured using the double-pour technique. This approach offers the best chance of pouring a master cast without distortion of the alginate. Since only a small amount of stone is added in the first pour, there is a minimum

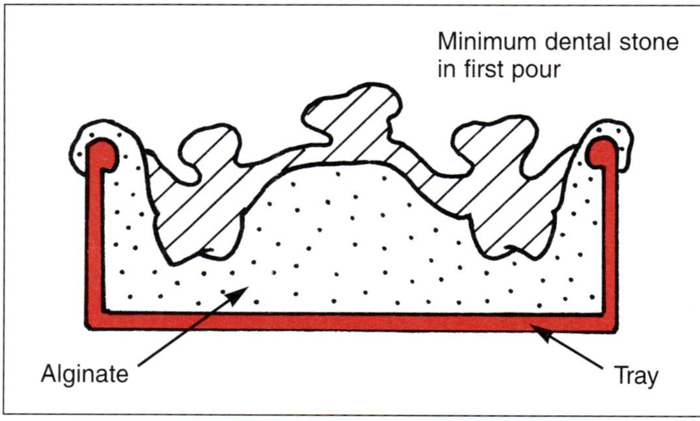

Fig 4-1 Cross section o⁻ ideal alginate with a minimum of 0.25 inch of impression material.

load placed on the alginate as compared to boxing and pouring the entire cast at one time. Once the stone has reached the initial set, the addition of the base presents no opportunity for distortion. The only potential problem arises when inadequate retentive blobs of stone are placed on the first pour (Fig 4-1). Without this retention, there is a possibility that the master cast will separate in the flask during boilout and flask opening.

If a vacuum mixing device is available to the operatory, the clinician can pour the first pour right at the chair and thereby assure that the impression has been correctly managed. The impression with the first pour should be placed in a humidor of some type for the initial set. The base can be added anytime thereafter. Die stone is indicated for the master cast, not for any increase in accuracy but for greater resistance to abrasion.

When the cast is recovered, it should be trimmed as soon as possible so that any blebs can be removed easily. When the cast is shaped with the model trimmer, a thin slurry inevitably covers the cast and, if it is not removed, will affect the accuracy of the cast. The slurry can be removed with a soft brush and running water; this should be done immediately. Dies or other critical areas can be protected from the slurry by covering them with a latex or silicone material before trimming the cast. The cast should be trimmed to the smallest possible dimension without compromising the critical areas. The smaller cast will allow a greater bulk of duplicating agar in the flask. Undercut areas, blebs, or other rough areas on the tongue side of the mandibular cast should be removed to reduce the possibility of tearing the agar. The distal extension edentulous areas that will require an altered cast tray should be clearly marked so that the technician will know exactly where the borders of the tray will end.

A final task that is unique to the maxillary master cast is that of beading the outline of the major connector. To reduce the tendency for food to impact beneath the major connector, a bead line is scraped into the cast following the outline. In general, a width of 1.5 mm and a depth of 1 mm will suffice to ensure a positive contact with the underlying soft tissue. The beading extends to within 4 to 6 mm from the marginal gingival tissues and there phases out completely. The bead line is to be rounded rather than sharp and is usually created with a discoid carver or a rounded curette.

The master cast must be resurveyed and, depending on the arrangement with the laboratory, the design of the framework neatly drawn. If the clinician is unable to make a precise drawing of the desired framework, it is better to leave the master cast unmarked and send the diagnostic cast as a reference for the technician along with the work authorization form. Work authorizations vary depending on custom and jurisdiction, but the more thorough the design and instructions, the greater the likelihood that the technician will be encouraged to return a casting of the highest quality.

For the most part, jaw relation records are made on the framework after it has been fitted to the mouth. There will be occasions when the master cast must be mounted before construction of the framework can begin. These situations always involve occlusion, especially when the space available for denture teeth is limited or when components of the framework must be in contact with opposing teeth. When anterior teeth are being replaced with the partial denture and a steep vertical overlap exists without any significant horizontal component, mounted master casts are essential.

Whenever possible, the master cast should be related to the opposing cast without the imposition of any recording material and the casts should be mounted by the clinician to assure accuracy. When insufficient teeth remain for positive positioning of the casts, a record base is constructed and a record made, usually in centric occlusion. The recording material should be completely plastic when the record is made and have a final set that is rigid. Bosworth's Superbite Paste (ZnO) or Blue Mousse are most often used. If the master cast is sent to the laboratory without being articulated, then witness lines are placed between teeth of the master cast and the opposing cast when the casts are in the desired occlusion. At least two marks per side are required to allow the technician to place the casts in the exact position. Any mounted cast must have had notches placed on the base of the cast to allow the cast to be repositioned on the mounting plaster, since the master cast will have to be removed for blockout and duplication.

The construction of a record base for a partial denture master cast is not without some risk of damaging the abutment stone teeth. A combination of wax blockout, plasticized polymethyl methacrylate (PMME), and autopolymerizing orthodontic resin (Dentsply/Caulk), used with the following technique, will permit the construction of an accurately fitting base without injury to the master cast.

First, the master cast is surveyed and soft tissue undercuts, if they exist, are identified by circling them with a pencil line. The outline of the desired record base is also drawn. It is not essential that the base contact all the remaining teeth, but some points of tooth contact are critical (at least three, widely spread when possible). A small amount of baseplate wax is flowed into the gingival crevice of the teeth to be contacted. Any undercuts in the denture base area greater than 3 mm are also blocked out with wax. The cast is then rehydrated by placing the base of the cast in water and allowing the moisture to penetrate the entire cast.

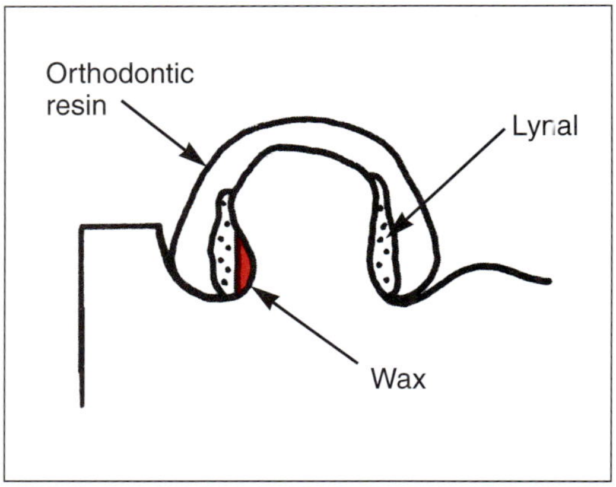

Fig 4-2 Blockout with wax and Lynal for sprinkle on base (cross section, lower midline).

The cast must not be submerged in water, as the accuracy of the tooth portions can be altered with the dissolution of the stone. Once the cast is hydrated, tinfoil substitute, diluted 2:1, is painted on. Caulk's Lynal or similar plasticized resin is added to any undercut areas and around the necks of the teeth that will be contacted by the record base. The Lynal is mixed thicker than is recommended by the manufacturer, to the consistency of peanut butter, so that it will stay where placed. Orthodontic resin is immediately added in a "salt and pepper technique" to complete the record base (Fig 4-2). The autopolymerizing resin will bond to the Lynal, and the resulting record base will be retained by the intrusion of the plasticized resin into the undercuts. There is no need to place the cast in the pressure pot for curing.

The base can be removed as soon as the resin is hard and trimmed. A wax rim can be added with the intent of having a supporting table of wax 2 to 3 mm out of occlusion. The recording material is mixed and placed on the table, and a centric record, at the desired occluding vertical dimension, is quickly made. The casts can be mounted on the articulator or submitted to the laboratory with the record for articulation. The laboratory technician can make a mounting record from the articulator to enable the mounting of the refractory cast to the opposing cast for the waxing of the occluding portions of the framework.

Altered Cast Impressions

Made only after the casting is finished, the altered cast impression is an attempt to combine the support of the abutment teeth with the support that can be obtained from the edentulous ridge. Originally, altered cast impressions were made on any edentulous area that had no posterior abutment, either maxillary or mandibular. Since the maxillary RPD is so well-supported by the major connector, little additional support is gained with an altered cast impression for a maxillary distal extension area, especially if the final impression was made in a custom tray. The difficulty of capturing the total denture space of the mandibular distal extension in the final impression has made the altered cast impression essential for all mandibular Class I and II situations. With the use of an altered cast impression, the clinician need not be overly concerned with the accuracy of the edentulous areas and can concentrate instead on making the best possible impression of the teeth to be contacted by the partial denture. It is essential that the full extent of the denture space in the distal extension of the edentulous ridge be captured so that the outline of the desired altered cast tray can be drawn as a part of the design. The technician can then return the framework with the altered cast tray in place, with its borders 2 to 3 mm short of the desired final extension of the denture base in the edentulous area.

The altered cast tray is constructed on the master cast after the casting has been completed. One thickness of baseplate wax, the same as for the relief for the retentive mesh, is adapted to the master cast to the outline of the desired altered cast tray extension. The retentive mesh area is heated over a Bunsen burner and the framework is seated onto the cast. The hot metal of the mesh must melt the relief wax and allow the casting to fully seat. With the tip of a spatula, the wax that extruded up through some of the mesh holes is removed to allow the resin of the tray to lock onto the framework. The tray resin is mixed and a small amount is removed from the mixing jar and immediately placed into the retentive holes that have been cleared of wax. The fluidity of this resin would not allow it to be used as yet to form the tray, but it will flow into the retentive areas easily and provide the required retention. The remainder of the tray resin is added when it is no longer tacky and the tray is formed. The tray must be kept to the dimensions of the ideal denture base. To form the ideal denture border, the tray must be uniformly short and be slightly undercontoured to make space for the impression material to capture the border without becoming bulky. When the occlusal portion of the tray is kept thin, it will occasionally be possible to make the final jaw relation record at the same appointment as the altered cast impression. If at that time the patient is unable to close the teeth into the desired occlusion for the record because of the thickness of the tray or the general lack of interocclusal space, the jaw registration must be made at a separate appointment.

The altered cast impression is made only after the framework has been fitted to the mouth and the full seating of the casting verified (the actual fitting of the frame will be discussed in Chapter 6). With the framework seated firmly on the abutment teeth, the extensions of the altered cast tray are evaluated. They are to be 2 to 3 mm short of the reflection of the border tissues. When the tray is properly extended, there is no need for border molding as a separate step. The wash impression will also give ideal borders if the tray is in the proper position relative to the tissues.

The choice of impression material to be used for this impression does not appear to be critical. Early studies indicated that mouth-temperature wax impressions placed the denture base tissues in their most supportive state. This material is seldom used because it requires a good deal of experience to read the quality of the impression. Polyether impression materials offer the option of varying the viscosity by blending high- and low-viscosity materials into one mix. The firmer the underlying tissue, the higher the percentage of high-viscosity impression material. When a good deal of unsupported soft tissue is found on the ridge crest, the mixture is altered to use a greater proportion of low-viscosity material. While a wash of all low-viscosity material will make an impression of this unsupported tissue with a minimum of pressure, it will tend to have poorly rounded borders because it is not thick enough to create the best border contours.

Excess saliva should be removed from the mouth, but there is no reason to have the mouth totally dry. The tray is loaded with just enough material to make up for the spacer, and an additional 20% is added to assure full border contours. There must be no excess material at the internal finishing line, as this material can flow up into the guide plate area when the frame is seated. When placing the framework in the mouth, the clinician must make sure that the frame is fully seated and that no pressure is placed on the tray itself. The fingers are placed on three widely separated rests to maintain the frame in its optimum position while the borders are developed and the material sets.

When fully set, the impression is removed from the mouth and trimmed to remove any excess impression material. There will normally be a thin extension of the material into the retromolar space on mandibular impressions and an extension of material onto the soft palate for the occasional maxillary impression. Since it is almost impossible to fully border mold the retromolar space on the altered cast tray, the determination of the extent of the resin border in this area is arbitrary. Remember that there is no need for full extension into the retromolar space in the removable partial denture as there would be for a complete denture. The retention of the partial denture is not dependent on this border. If a large undercut exists distal to the mylohyoid ridge, the denture base may be prohibited from entering the undercut, as it might in a complete denture, since the guiding planes determine the path of insertion. It is acceptable for the lingual extension of the flange to terminate at the soft tissue height of contour as determined by these guiding planes. The patient will be more comfortable with less resin in the mouth, and the support of the extension base will not be compromised, since it is the ridge crest and the external oblique ridge that are the supporting structures for the distal extension.

Any borders of insufficient width can be recreated in wax if they are extended to the predetermined limits. Since this border width is arbitrary in the removable partial denture, there is no need to confirm the width in the patient's mouth at this time. Should excess wax flow onto the internal surface of the impression when the borders are being created, it can easily be removed without damaging the accuracy of the impression.

A final verification of the distal extension impression must be made after the base is trimmed and shaped. At this time the clinician must be confident that the frame fully seats and that all impression material that has flowed onto the framework has been removed. Special consideration must be given to removing any material that extends beyond the internal finishing line. A sharp blade should be used to trim the material in this area so that no pulling or tearing of the impression material occurs. At this point a jaw relation record can be made if required and if adequate space for the record exists.

Pouring the altered cast impression can be delegated to the technician, but the clinician must verify that the framework is fully seated on the master cast and that sticky wax has been added to hold the cast and frame together during the boxing and pouring of the stone. This means that the original edentulous portion of the master cast must have been removed earlier and that adequate retention has been cut into the remainder of the master cast. Rather than go through an elaborate boxing process, the clinician may elect to pour the altered cast impression in two stages, much as was done for the master cast. The border roll of the altered cast impression must be preserved in the boxing and pouring of the impression. A line is drawn on the impression with an indelible marker just at the point where the border contour is complete. Boxing material is placed at this line to create a land area of 3 mm, the impression is filled with vacuum-mixed stone, and retentive blobs are placed (Fig 4-3). The base can be added later, after the initial set, without fear of disturbing the tooth-frame relation. The altered cast impression is poured in standard yellow stone rather than in the same die stone as was used for the original master cast. The softer yellow stone is far easier than die stone to remove from the processed denture base with the use of the walnut shell blaster and stone solvent.

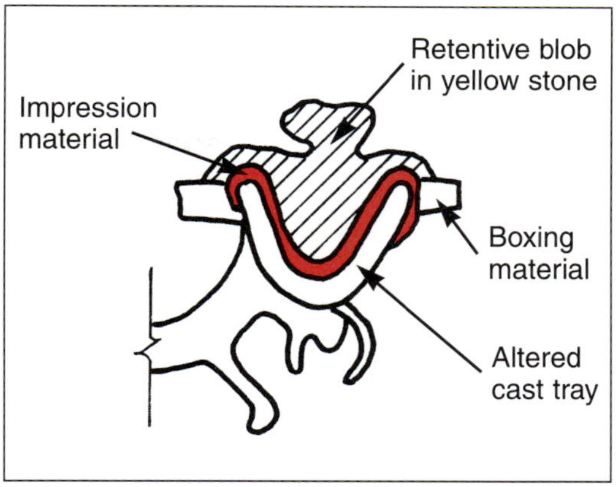

Fig 4-3 Double pour for altered cast impression (base is added later).

Jaw Relation Records

When sufficient interocclusal space exists, it makes sense to make the jaw relation record before pouring the altered cast impression, thus saving the patient an additional visit. The recording material of choice is again one that is completely plastic to start and that sets hard quickly. The occluding surface of the tray is prepared by cutting a few crossing grooves in the resin or, when a great deal of space exists, adding a wax occlusion rim to reduce the space for the recording material. Since there will be natural teeth in contact in all dentate cases, only a very small amount of recording material need be placed. Three well-defined and widely separated points of positive contact will allow accurate articulation of the casts. Once the stone has set and the base completed and trimmed, the cast with the framework and tray in position is articulated with the opposing cast and mounted in the articulator before the impression is separated from the cast. When the opposing arch is a complete denture, the jaw relation records are made at a separate appointment since there are other procedures that must be completed as a part of this patient treatment.

No compromise in the quality of the final impression or master cast can be allowed. The clinician must be prepared, and must prepare the patient, for the inevitable remakes that will occur. Once patients understand that only perfection is acceptable at this critical stage, they will see that it is in their best interests to cooperate fully. In addition, technicians must feel comfortable in telling clinicians that an apparent error has been identified on the master cast. Their advice must always be welcomed, even though the natural reaction to the requested remake is one of irritation. It is through this team approach that partials of the highest quality are made on a routine basis.

5

Laboratory Construction of the Framework

The laboratory phase of removable partial denture construction is just as important as the clinical phase. Because of the expensive equipment required to cast stellate alloys, the clinician is totally dependent on the dental technician to construct the framework. As a result of this situation, dental schools do not prepare their students to make frameworks and, unless the clinician has had laboratory experience before dental school, he or she will understand the procedures necessary to create quality frameworks only in the most basic sense. Nonetheless, the clinician bears the ultimate responsibility for the quality of the prostheses placed in the mouth and so must carefully interface with the laboratory to maintain this standard.

Clinicians have, unfortunately, often used the laboratory as a scapegoat for problems that arise during treatment. Problems in clinic-laboratory relations can most often be traced to lack of communication and the unwillingness of the clinician to review the laboratory procedures at the appropriate stages in construction. For example, the clinician should always have the blocked-out master cast and the waxed-up refractory cast returned for evaluation before spruing and casting the framework. This evaluation is well worth the delay it presents, as there will always be cases for which the clinician is unable to adequately describe what is desired in the final product. The interaction between the clinician and the technician is equally significant for fixed prosthodontic restorations in the situations described in Chapter 3 in the discussion of additive mouth preparation.

The phases of RPD construction in the laboratory can be divided into:

- Design transfer
- Blockout and duplication
- Waxing
- Spruing, investing, and casting
- Metal finishing
- Addition of wire clasps (where indicated)
- Addition of the altered cast tray (where indicated)

The actual construction techniques and

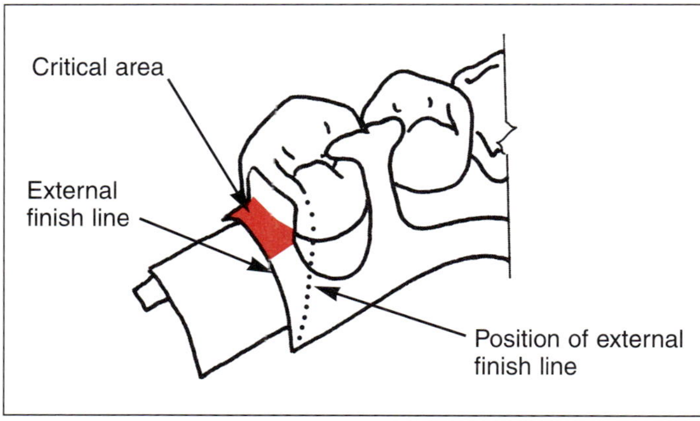

Fig 5-1 Placement of internal finish line.

materials are usually proprietary, having been developed by the dental laboratory industry and the metal manufacturing companies. The alloys are generally chrome based, although iron and titanium alloys have been proposed and are in use. Vitallium and Ticonium are the most commonly used commercial alloys in North America. These two alloys use different investments and different duplicating agars but are otherwise quite similar in their construction techniques. They show similar results in materials testing as well. The composition and characteristics of these alloys are available in any text on dental materials and should be a part of the knowledge base of the clinician involved with prosthodontics at the advanced level.

Design Transfer

Construction in the laboratory begins with the transfer of the design from the diagnostic cast or the work authorization to the master cast. Specialists who are comfortable with their ability to make a precise drawing on the master cast need to be sure that the color code they employ is known to the technician. By placing the design on the tripoded master cast, one area of potential error is eliminated. Special care must be taken in the outline of relief pads for retentive meshwork. The extent of the internal finishing line must be clearly marked 1.5 to 2 mm from the gingival marginal tissue so that this area will be in metal rather than in resin (Fig 5-1). Heights of contour must be carefully marked with the surveyor lead on both hard and soft tissues so that no areas requiring blockout are missed.

Perhaps the most critical area of design transfer is the accurate drawing of retentive clasp arms. The terminal third of all circumferential cast clasps must be accurately placed at the desired undercut depth, almost always 0.010 inch (0.250 mm). Depending on the steepness of the undercut and the amount of mouth preparation, undercuts in the terminal third of the tooth surface may require blockout even though ideally the entire terminal third of the clasp should be contacting the tooth in the undercut area. A master cast must be rejected if the available undercuts are inadequate in depth or position on the tooth. Before deciding that the master cast will not be acceptable, the path of insertion/removal must be reviewed to assure that the cast is, in fact, at the proper tilt on the surveyor.

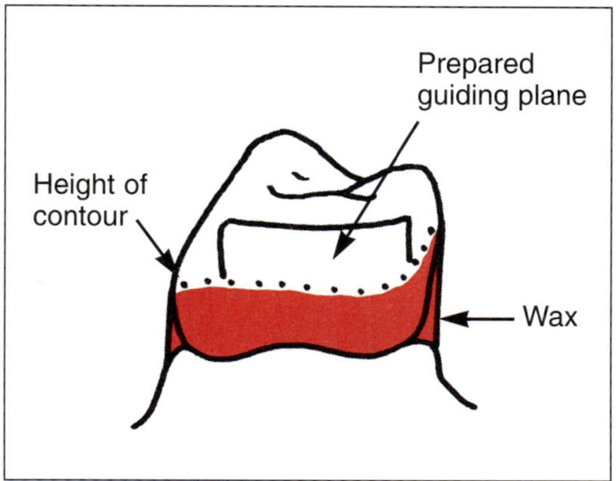

Fig 5-2 Relation of guiding plane and blockout wax.

Blockout and Duplication

Depending on the proprietary techniques specific to the alloy being used for the framework, the designed master cast may be sprayed with a model gloss to seal the cast and preserve the drawn design. Obviously, care must be taken not to overspray since any accumulation of the protective coating would change the dimensions of the master cast and may result in an unusable casting. Most modern techniques have eliminated this process.

Blockout wax, either the commercially available blends or homemade, is then placed on the stone teeth to begin the blockout process. It is essential that no blockout wax be placed above the line indicating the height of contour on any areas where the casting is intended to touch the teeth, on guiding planes, rest seats, and clasp arms (Fig 5-2). The reason for stressing this seemingly benign step is that the contours of the stone teeth will inevitably be changed by the process in areas where accuracy is essential to the final fit of the casting. The technician removes the excess blockout wax using a vertical blade in a surveying instrument, sometimes even one that is electrically heated, to increase the possibility of creating a smooth surface on the refractory cast. Wax placed above the height of contour in areas of tooth-frame contact must also be removed. In an attempt to do so, the technician will either leave a small amount of wax, thereby making the master cast and resultant refractory slightly larger than it really is, or, in attempting to remove all the excess wax, scrape some of the stone and thereby make the master cast slightly smaller in that area. In either situation, the accuracy of the master cast has been compromised. It is far better to be very careful in the initial placement of the blockout wax and never have to deal with the problems that arise in its removal.

The blockout is generally done at 0 degrees, parallel with the intended path of insertion/removal. It is possible to alter this angle by substituting a blade that has a 2- or 6-degree angle. This type of divergent blockout is used primarily for certain types of precision attachment situations. In using a blockout of other than 0 degrees, frictional resistance to dislodgment is inevitably lost, forcing increased reliance on clasp retention.

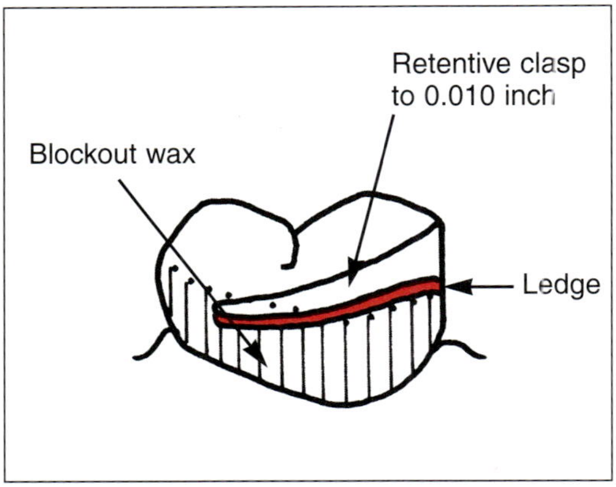

Fig 5-3 Blockout ledge for clasp placement.

Some laboratories use a technique in which a ledge is created in the blockout wax at the inferior border of clasp arms. This ledge is duplicated in the refractory and serves as a shelf onto which the plastic clasp pattern is placed during the wax-up. It should be obvious that the ledge must be placed with careful regard for the underlying drawing of the clasp arm (Fig 5-3). Since the placement of the plastic clasp pattern to a precise position on the refractory cast is not an easy task, the ledge should be placed slightly (about 0.5 mm) below the line that represents the inferior border of the clasp. This will ensure that the clasp will reach the desired undercut position.

When the abutment teeth have been recontoured with the blockout wax to the extent prescribed, the relief pads are added to the master cast. A full thickness of baseplate wax (roughly 1 mm) is the minimum for the relief of the retentive mesh. Commercial laboratories often choose to use a thinner relief wax in the belief that keeping the meshwork closer to the edentulous areas creates more room for the rapid placement of the denture teeth. While this is true, a relief pad that is too thin creates insufficient space for quality resin under the meshwork as well as an internal finishing line that does not have adequate depth to retain the resin in the critical area next to the abutment tooth. The relief pad thickness also determines the amount of space that will be available for the impression material of the altered cast impression. Again, 1 mm is the minimum space for impression. In addition, the recommended procedure for a reline of the distal extension base involves first removing a uniform amount of material to ensure a good bond of the added resin to the old denture base. When less than a millimeter of resin exists under the meshwork, the reduction of the material often results in grinding completely through to the mesh. The thickness of the relief wax pad must be prescribed by the clinician, not determined arbitrarily by the laboratory, especially where overdenture abutments and implants are involved (to be discussed later). The relief pad must be sealed to the master cast so that it does not separate in the duplicating procedures to follow.

To complete the blockout procedures, wax or caulking materials are placed in all undercuts that are not part of the framework. Blockout of these nonessential areas is important, nonetheless, since the entire cast must be removed from the duplicating mold without tearing the agar. Any undercuts other than the 0.010 inch for the clasp retention have the potential to distort the agar. The fully blocked-out cast is placed in a saturated solution of dental stone to be hydrated before duplicating it in the refractory material.

The duplicating agar is commonly one that is provided by the manufacturer of the alloy system and is chosen for compatibility with the refractory material. For example, a phosphate-bonded investment does not set against a water-based colloid, so a glycerin-based duplicating agar is used for the higher-heat alloys. The agar is usually kept in an electrically heated dispenser, from which it is poured through a controlled valve into the duplicating flask at a prescribed temperature and to which it is returned after recovery from the set refractory at the end of the duplicating process. The duplicating material does have an expiration point based on the number of times it has been broken down and reheated. Clinicians need only assure themselves that the laboratory does indeed record the number of cycles and replaces the agar at the appropriate times as directed by the manufacturer.

The flask used to contain the duplicating agar is designed with a metal base and a nonmetallic side ring that fits into a channel on the base. The blocked-out master cast is placed on the base, and the hot (temperature depending on manufacturer) agar is slowly poured into the flask up to the level of the top of the ring. The entire flask is placed into a circulating cold-water bath, where the metal of the base conducts the shrinkage of the cooling agar toward the base to result in an accurate mold. When the agar is cooled to room temperature, the flask is removed from the bath. The master cast is carefully removed from the mold by placing a knife blade in the cast base at both sides and lifting the cast vertically out of the mold without stressing the agar. Having the sides of the base of the master cast trimmed to diverge slightly toward the base will make removal easier.

The liquid-powder ratio for the refractory cast is critical for the accuracy of the casting. The density of the set refractory determines, to a great extent, the expansion of the investment mold. It has been claimed that a change as little as 1 cc of liquid in the liquid-powder ratio can affect the clinical fit of the framework. Because of the high casting temperatures of the stellate alloys, the thermal shrinkage with cooling is significant. Our ability to sufficiently expand the mold is limited. By decreasing the amount of liquid to powder, the expansion of the mold can be increased to offset the thermal shrinkage. Unfortunately, the thickening of the mix that results from the change in the ratio makes the mass too thick to pour into the agar mold without fear of trapping air. The technician who uses the manufacturer's recommended ratio with exact measurements of both liquid and powder will generally produce a mold with adequate expansion. Beware of the technician who is careless with the measurement of the liquid or perhaps overlooks water in the bottom of the mixing bowl. A mix that has too much liquid in the ratio results in a mold that cannot expand sufficiently to match the expected thermal shrinkage.

Most techniques for the casting of these RPD alloys call for the desiccation of the refractory cast in an oven to remove excess moisture, followed by dipping the cast in a bath of hot molten beeswax. This wax seals the pores of the refractory and makes it less susceptible to abrasion. It also eliminates the need to soak the refractory cast before adding the first layer of paint-on investment over the waxed framework. Commercial model spray can also be used for these purposes. Two light coats of spray are required, with a 2- to 3-minute drying time between coats.

Waxing

At this point, the design is again transferred, from the master cast to the refractory cast, to form the outline for the waxing of the framework. The clinician has every right to expect a casting that conforms to the design placed on the master cast. Commercially available plastic patterns are used whenever possible to maintain standard dimensions for major connectors, clasps, and finishing lines. Rests are apt to be hand-waxed to blend in with the plastic patterns. The clinician needs to have seen the patterns and evaluated their shape and thickness to be able to truly prescribe the components of the framework. Because clasp patterns have such a major effect on the performance of the cast clasp and come in such a variety of tapers and width-thickness ratios, they must be selected with care.

The plastic patterns are quite flexible and can easily be stretched when removing them from the cards on which they come or when adapting them to the refractory cast. They also have a memory, so they must be held in place with some sort of adhesive that is compatible with the entire process. A mixture of acetone and the plastic pattern material will create a tacky liquid that can be painted onto the refractory and to which the patterns will adhere. The tacky liquid should have only enough viscosity to glue the pattern in place. Excess material painted on the cast will result in a change in dimension of the resultant casting.

Once the tacky liquid has been applied, the patterns are cut to length, and occasionally shape, and adapted with either finger pressure or with a soft pencil eraser (or similar instrument). Sharp instruments may create cuts or grooves in the patterns that may influence the performance of the final casting. The sections of the plastic patterns will have to be joined with wax, trying to maintain the contours of the pattern. Since the resultant casting will not come out of the casting process as smooth and precise as a cast crown, the wax is always added in slight excess to allow for finishing and polishing of the surface. Where clasp arms join the minor connectors, care must be taken to assure that the taper established will not create a thin area in the active portion of the clasp or at the junction of the plastic pattern and the minor connector which will often be thinner than the pattern (Fig 5-4). This thin area, in between two thicker areas, can only act to concentrate stress, and, thus, a fractured clasp can be predicted in the future.

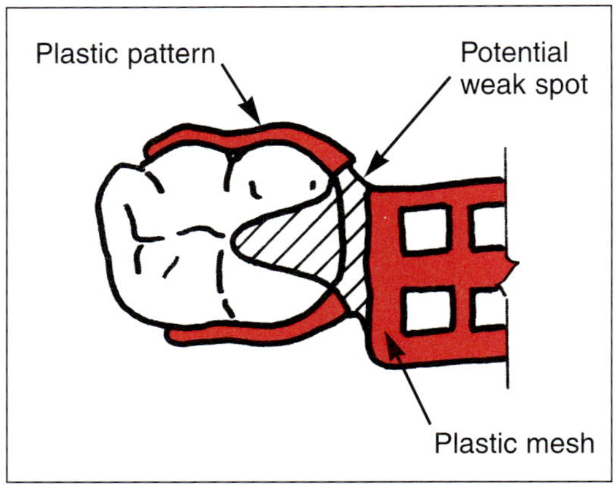

Fig 5-4 Junction of plastic pattern and hand-waxed minor connector.

The blockout/relief pad established the internal finish line, so the technician need only worry about the accurate placement of the external finish line. This line, usually a portion of a plastic pattern, should extend to the occlusal portion of the line angle of the abutment (Fig 5-5). This position will

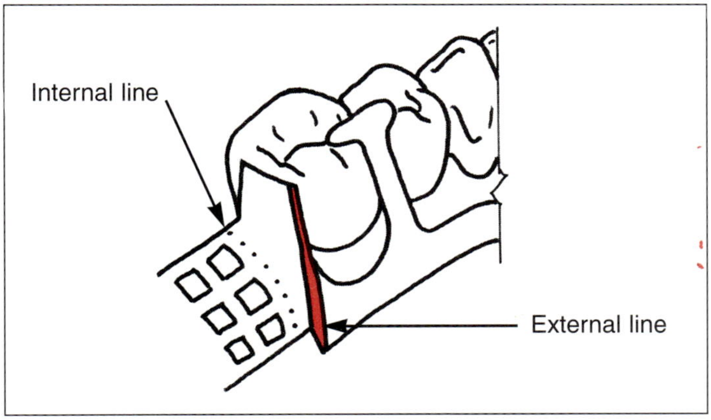

Fig 5-5 Placement of external finish line.

permit a small amount of denture base resin between the denture tooth and the casting in the completed prosthesis.

The tips of cast clasp patterns should extend to just beyond the terminal extension of the transferred design to allow a small excess of metal, no more than 0.5 mm, for finishing.

Distal extension meshwork will require a tissue stop to be added at the end of the relief area of the refractory, either distal or mesial depending on the situation. The stop should be roughly 3 × 3 mm and should be placed on the crest of the edentulous ridge or slightly buccal to it, wherever a relatively flat area can be found. The stop indicates a complete seating of the casting in that area for fitting and finishing. It will be removed as part of the altered cast procedure in situations where this type of impression is required.

While the plastic pattern of the meshwork is adequate for the vast majority of situations, there are occasions when the resin retention should be created freehand in wax. Loops or strips of one-half round 8- or 10-gauge wax can be placed on the relief area of the refractory and waxed into the finish line area. This approach is most effective for maxillary tuberosity areas, where space for resin is at a premium. The larger retentive areas of the hand-waxed resin retention may create a stronger link to the processed resin, although the shape of the commercial patterns appears to be adequate. However, the patterns do not provide adequate retention for resin in constricted spaces. Should mesh be required in the space of a single tooth, custom waxing of the retention is desirable because the small lattice arrangement of the plastic patterns will not provide sufficient retention.

At this point, the refractory cast and the blocked-out master cast are to be returned to the clinician for review. It is essential that this review take place for every case until the technician truly understands the quality level expected by the clinician. For complex cases and all precision attachment partials, it must be standard practice. The technician sees that the clinician cares about quality and is knowledgeable about laboratory techniques. Misunderstandings that inevitably occur on design and construction are most often the fault of the clinician being unable to describe in words exactly what is required. It is only common sense that the wax-up should be reviewed before spruing and investing. It has been my experience that some aspect of the wax-up will need to be refined in about 25% of cases, and that percentage makes the inconvenience worthwhile.

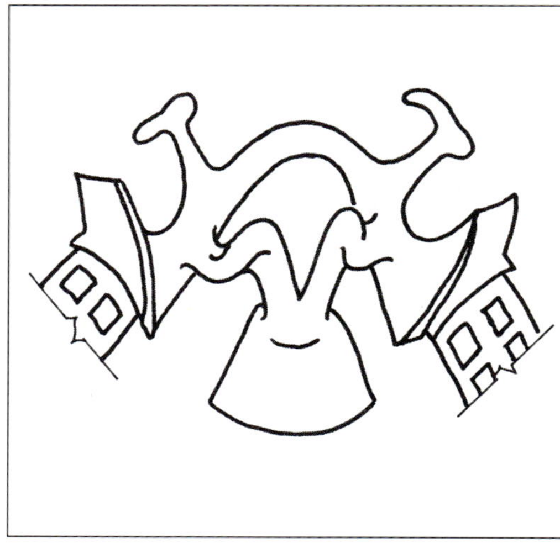

Fig 5-6 Helical sprue leads reduce turbulence.

Spruing, Investing, and Casting

These steps in the laboratory construction of the removable partial denture are industrial in nature and generally follow the proprietary instructions of the metal manufacturer. The clinician does not have a role to play here except for being aware of the process, especially the spruing, since the variation in spruing techniques is great—with every technician doing things a bit differently. As an example, the laboratory with which I have worked for 18 years uses a helix in the sprue leads, usually two or three leads for a mandibular casting and four for a maxillary (Fig 5-6). The technicians feel that the helix does two things that dramatically affect the quality of the casting: *(1)* it acts as a reservoir for the metal mass that reduces the potential of a suckback, and *(2)* it slows the flow of the molten metal, however briefly, reducing the turbulence and thus reducing porosity. Sprue leads without the helix are sometimes used as an additional lead for complex casting configurations. These sprues are always slightly curved to slow the metal flow.

The clinician should always examine the resultant casting and any broken castings for evidence of porosity as a quality-control check on the laboratory. It is possible, but not practical, to x-ray a casting using an occlusal film to visualize porosity, as was standard practice for subperiosteal implants.

While there is little that the clinician can do, beyond showing interest, about the casting of the partial denture framework, the treatment of the casting after it has been cast is a critical procedure that dramatically affects the ultimate success of the partial denture.

Metal Finishing

Metal finishing is an all-encompassing term covering the steps from the actual casting of the partial denture framework to the fully finished and polished framework. It is an aspect of the process that historically has been left entirely to the discretion of the technician, with the clinician accepting the finished product without question. The finishing and fitting of the casting is the most important phase of construction, and it is here where an accurate casting can easily be rendered unacceptable if the internal surfaces that contact the teeth are altered in any way. The standard means of finishing the casting, once the sprue(s) has been removed with a cut-off disc, is to electropolish, that is, strip the entire casting electronically in order to remove a small amount of metal from the entire surface. This process reduces the amount of fine finishing and polishing that will be required. Unfortunately, the removal of even this potentially very small amount of metal (40 to 50 microns) will reduce the frictional retention that could have been obtained with the parallel guiding planes established through mouth preparation. The only way to control this electrochemical process is to not allow it to occur at all.

All tooth-contacting surfaces—guide plates, minor connectors, rests, and clasps—must be protected from the electrolytic deplating process by coating them with a high-fusing wax or a substance such as fingernail polish that will not allow contact with the acid bath. Stripping or deplating occurs when a metal is placed in an acid bath attached to an electrode and a controlled microamperage is passed through the metal via the electrodes and the bath. A commercial unit with temperature and amperage control and timer, which has a clamp on the electrode to hold the framework, is used. Obviously, all the ingredients of the system contribute to the rate of dissolution of the surface of the framework and so are susceptible to improperly calibrated components or careless technicians. This system works in reverse as compared to a die-plating unit and is similar to the units used for microetching of bonded castings.

Once the contact surfaces have been protected, the frame can be safely placed in the bath and kept there until the normal dark color of the as-cast alloy is replaced by a clean and shiny surface. The frame is now ready for preliminary finishing and fitting to the cast. Once again, the clinician must demand that the contact surfaces are not touched in any way by the technician and that no fitting of the frame to the master cast take place in the laboratory. The technician is instructed to finish and polish the framework in a standard fashion, leaving the fitting to the clinician. The reason for stressing this point is that the technician, in attempting to fit the frame to the master cast, will inevitably remove more metal from the contact surfaces than is required, which decreases the quality of the tooth-frame relationship. Once a casting has been placed on a cast, the cast surface will be abraded and no longer accurate, so that subsequent fitting will be done to a cast that does not represent the mouth.

If the casting is not fitted to the master cast in the laboratory, then this responsibility will rest with the clinician. The state-of-the-art casting will first be fitted to the teeth by the clinician, and only when an acceptable relationship has been obtained will the casting be placed on the master cast. Should the cast be scraped in the process, it is not a concern because this will not affect the tooth-frame relationship. If it is not possible to fully seat the casting in the mouth, the master cast must be remade because there is no way to accurately determine if the cause of the misfit is an inaccurate impression or a laboratory error.

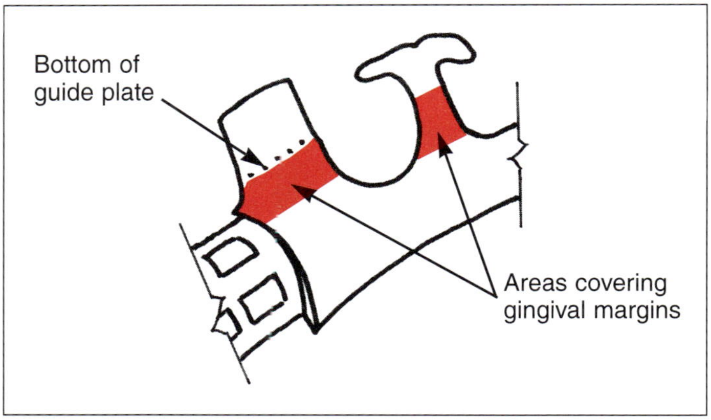

Fig 5-7 Internal view of casting, indicating areas requiring high polish.

The laboratory must be instructed to place the highest-possible finish on the casting gingival to the contact area of the guide plate (Fig 5-7). This will require careful use of stones and rubber wheels so as not to abrade the contact areas. This quality finish is required, since plaque retention in this area has the greatest potential for tissue damage. In fact, this is the only area of the partial denture for which there is a physiologic reason for polishing. All other surfaces could just as well be left in the as-cast state, except that the technician, clinician, and patient expect the appliance to be highly polished, as this is the customary finish for anything that goes into the mouth.

The clinician has two options for seating the casting on the master cast when the framework requires the additional steps of adding wire clasps or altered cast trays: *(1)* the casting can be returned to the clinician for the fitting of the frame and the fitted casting sent back to the laboratory on the master cast, or *(2)* the technician can be instructed to place the finished casting on the master cast in the lab, always at the expense of the stone teeth. The intraoral fitting of the framework can be done just as easily with the wires and the tray in place.

Addition of Wire Clasps

While it is technically possible to cast to wires, this procedure is primarily used for gold base castings and high–gold-content wires. When stellate alloys are used for the framework, the wire is best soldered to the finished framework some distance from the point of flexure. Casting a stellate alloy to a wire clasp or soldering the clasp directly to the minor connector will result in a brittle and more rigid clasp and increase the likelihood of subsequent clasp failure.

Wires for retentive clasp arms are most often round in cross section. It is possible, however, to use a half round clasp wire. There is no clinical evidence that this form has any advantage over the simpler shape. In fact, the half round wire is much more difficult to adapt to the tooth; any bend across the flat surface is a technical challenge. The desired position relative to the

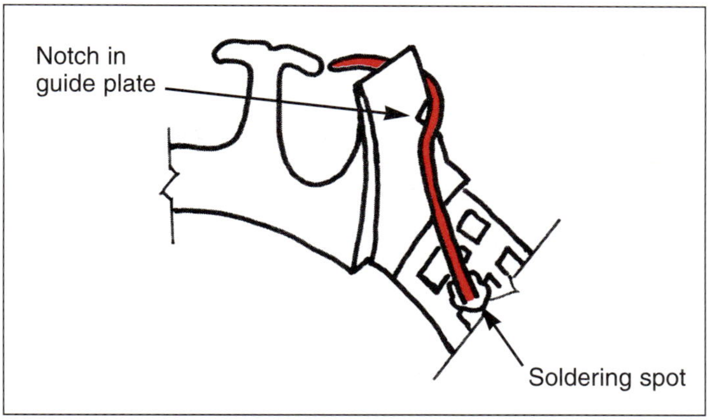

Fig 5-8 Position of wire clasp on framework.

height of contour has been indicated on the master cast and marked with a single line. The technician should be able to contour the wire exactly to this line. For the wire I-bar, the clinician must indicate just how much of the foot of the clasp should contact the tooth. Usually a gentle bend 2 to 3 mm from the tip of the clasp will give sufficient linear contact to ensure a positive contact of clasp on tooth. The tips of either form of wire clasp should be rounded before soldering them to the framework, since access to the tip may be limited once the clasp is in place.

The wire clasp is adapted to the master cast with the framework in place. Occasionally the guide plate is notched at the point where a circumferential clasp will exit the resin so the clasp can be positioned exactly as designed. The tang of the clasp is directed down the guide plate and onto the lingual surface of the casting. It will terminate in a positive contact area, either a retentive mesh square that has been filled in during the wax-up or a retentive bead that has been flattened with a disc after casting (Fig 5-8). In either instance, the wire must make a positive contact with the casting if resistance brazing is to be used to solder the clasp. Our studies have shown that an 800 fine solder will produce the best joints when used in conjunction with a non-precious or a PGP (platinum, gold, and palladium) wire. Softer wires (such as the Jelenko Standard Clasp Wire) are better soldered with a torch and conventional 650 solder.

Resistance brazing, which utilizes a step-down transformer and a carbon tip to heat the solder while a copper tip completes the circuit through the casting, is a quick means of soldering stellate alloys and is used extensively for repairing partial denture frameworks (Fig 5-9). Like all soldering operations, the brazing is an art rather than a science and considerable experience is required to create a dependable joint. Fortunately, the wire will also be retained by the resin, but to do this, the portion of the wire embedded in the denture base must have some bends for physical retention.

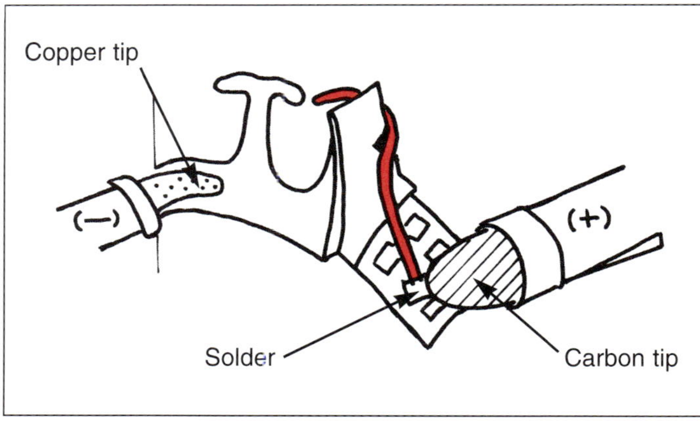

Fig 5-9 Resistance brazing to attach wire clasp to frame.

Addition of Altered Cast Trays

Mandibular distal extensions will require a secondary impression to relate the support of the soft tissue to that of the hard through the framework. As stated previously, certain maxillary situations will also require a secondary impression. The goal in the construction of these trays is to make a tray to a given outline of standard thickness and with adequate retention to the frame. All sharp areas must be rounded and any relief wax completely removed so that the tray can be immediately placed in the mouth without the need for alteration. The borders must be uniformly short of the desired final denture base extensions so that the altered cast impression can be satisfactorily made on the first attempt. It is reasonable to expect that if the clinician clearly outlines the desired extension of the trays and prescribes the thickness desired, these trays will conform to the work authorization.

While not as important as the maintenance of the hard and soft tissues of the oral cavity in the long term, the quality of the laboratory phases of construction dictates much of the potential for success of the removable partial denture. Finding the state-of-the-art dental laboratory and building a working relationship with the technicians will always be a major factor in the treatment of patients needing a removable partial denture. The more complex the partial, the greater the need for technicians to be fully involved in the process.

6

Establishing the Tooth-Frame Relationship

Since the laboratory technician has not touched the tooth contact areas of the framework during the recovery and finishing procedures, the responsibility for fitting the frame devolves entirely on the clinician. While this may be interpreted by some as unnecessary and time-consuming, there is no other way to obtain the highest-quality fit of the casting and to retain the frictional fit of the guide plates on the prepared guiding planes.

There are three phases of this fitting procedure: *(1)* correcting tooth contact surfaces, *(2)* obtaining static fit in the mouth, and *(3)* establishing a functional fit.

Tooth Contact Surfaces

Since the as-cast surface of a stellate casting is quite rough due to the porosity and grain size of the refractory, the first step is to examine the casting under magnification and to carefully remove all the blebs on the tooth contact surfaces, primarily the guide plates. Because the stellate alloys are so much harder than gold alloys, the adjustment of the contact spots is not easily or quickly accomplished. Special burs are available for these alloys. (The Brasseler Company makes an E-series bur for the straight handpiece intended to run at 10,000 to 15,000 rpm. These burs come in a variety of sizes and in both regular and fine cut. There are also fully sintered diamond stones that are intended for use with chrome alloys.) The goal at this point is to remove the positive imperfections without changing the contact surface of the guide plate. Once the blebs have been removed, the contact surfaces are sandblasted to leave a uniform matte surface to make the identification of intraoral contact points easier.

Static Fit

The second step in the fitting procedure is to obtain a static fit in the mouth, whereby the casting fully seats on the prepared teeth. Using magnifying loops and a sharp explorer, this fit is verified visually. The seating process begins with the use of a disclosing material to identify areas of premature contact. Historically, disclosing waxes or a mixture of gold rouge in chloroform was used to identify these areas. Both have been discontinued—the waxes because they were a mess to apply and to clean up and the chloroform-rouge mixture because of concerns related to the volatility of the chemical and its toxic nature. A convenient substitute has been found in Fit Checker, a GC product. This very thin and quick-setting silicone, intended for evaluating the fit of crowns, works equally well for frameworks. It identifies contact points in a static fit only, since it sets chemically.

For the casting that is difficult to seat, it is good to remember those areas most apt to be in hypercontact. Our studies have shown that the area most likely to have contact is at the marginal ridge, where the transition from the guide plate to the rest occurs. If the tooth preparation has left a sharp line angle here, chances are excellent that the cause of the casting not seating can be traced to this area. Unfortunately, identification with the Fit Checker in this area is not as obvious as it is on the flat surfaces of the guide plate. It is always possible that there are still some minor blebs at this critical junction that were not identified in the first step.

Functional Fit

Once a satisfactory static fit is obtained, usually after a number of adjustments of the guide plate surfaces, the fitting of the frame is complete for all but Class I partial dentures. For the bilateral free-end situation, functional relief is required if the clinician wants the supporting areas of the edentulous ridges to bear some of the load of mastication. Remember, if no functional stress relief is created in the casting, either through the short guiding plane concept already discussed or the use of tapered blockout, the casting must be relieved to allow some rotation movement around the distalmost points of contact.

How much stress relief is desirable? There is no clear scientific answer to this question. It may be best to tailor the amount of movement to the displacement of the areas of major support for the denture bases. When the ridge tissue is firm and healthy, little relief is needed to protect the abutment teeth from luxation. However, when the supporting tissues are weaker, the amount of possible base movement in function is increased and the amount of stress relief must be increased. As a general rule, if 2 mm of rotational movement is possible at the distal extension of the retentive mesh without binding on the abutment teeth, stress relief will have been established. The longer the edentulous span, the greater the amount of stress relief that must be created in the casting.

To rotate the framework, the tissue stop must be removed from the distal extension of the meshwork. If it is not removed, it will, quite possibly, dig into the soft tissue beneath it and restrict rotational movement. Next, a small square of Mylar-based articulating ribbon (Accu-Film II or similar material) is cut and placed in the casting in the area of the guide plate. This material is generally about 30 microns thick, not enough to have any effect on the procedure. The casting is seated and rotated by placing a vertical load on the distalmost part of the meshwork or the altered cast tray (if one is attached at this point). The die incorporated in the Mylar ribbon transfers easily to both casting and tooth to identify the areas of heavy contact with rotation. The casting is adjusted, always with care not to remove any more metal than is absolutely necessary, until the desired movement is obtained. The Mylar has just enough elasticity to adapt itself around the tooth. It, and the tooth, must be completely dry to lay down a crisp mark at the point of contact.

The combination of parallel or "milled" guiding planes, accurate final impression, and attention to detail in the laboratory should create a casting that can be fully seated without eliminating the frictional resistance to removal of the framework. Even the finest casting can be severely compromised by careless fitting of the frame. The clinician must get in the habit of treating the partial denture casting with the same care as would be given to a crown margin.

What should one do if the framework does not completely seat on the abutment teeth? In some instances it may be possible to retrofit the casting to the abutment tooth by bonding on resin to contact the frame. The most obvious example of retrofitting is when the casting fits everywhere except for one or two rests that fail to contact their rest seats. When these rest seats are in enamel it is both convenient and acceptable to etch the existing rest seat, prime the enamel with any suitable bonding agent, and then place composite resin on the rest area and seat the framework. In most instances, sufficient light can be transferred to the composite by varying the angle of the light source to achieve a stable mass of resin. Excess material that may have extruded over the casting is eliminated and the framework is removed. Additional light curing is done before any finishing procedures are undertaken. The quality of fit of the new rest seat will be perfect because the seat was made to fit the existing casting. Other areas of the framework are not as easy to retrofit, but using chemically cured composites, guiding planes can be brought into contact with the guide plate. Our recent studies have shown a dramatic increase in frictional retention with these retrofitted contacts. These composite retrofits have stood up remarkably well over an 8- to 10-year period.

In addition to fitting the frame to the teeth, the frame must also be brought into occlusal harmony with the natural teeth. The clinician must evaluate the natural tooth stops without the partial casting in the mouth and assure that the presence of the casting has not altered this relationship. Since the occlusal and incisal rests are routinely overcontoured in the wax-up, it is to be expected that on some occasions the cast metal may well interfere with complete closure to centric occlusion. The clinician should first evaluate the thickness of the offending rest by measuring, both at the center of the rest and at the marginal ridge area, the thickness of the metal. The rest should never be reduced beyond 1.2 mm for fear of subsequent fracture, sometimes months or years later. When this dimension is reached, further adjustment must be done on the opposing tooth. Obviously, careful mouth preparation will reduce the need for these adjustments.

Since the occlusal surface of the rest will have to be finished with rubber wheels and polished after adjustment, the metal should be sandblasted on those surfaces to make the identification of the die marks from the Accu-Film easier to spot. It is not easy to return the laboratory finish to the casting with standard chairside finishing stones and rubber points. The hardness of the metal requires that a high-speed dental lathe be used to quickly restore the metal to its original luster. The repolishing of these occluding surfaces is a laboratory function and should be completed before the positioning on the denture teeth begins.

The additional time and effort required to establish the ideal tooth-frame relationship must be added to the total cost of creating the very finest partial dentures. Without this level of attention to the final fit, the goals of esthetic tooth replacement without visible anterior clasping and the substitution of frictional retention for clasp retention cannot be achieved on a routine basis. As the partial denture becomes more sophisticated with the addition of precision attachments and implants, the ability to control the interface becomes even more essential to creating partial dentures of the highest quality.

Poor Casting Fit

Inevitably, the clinician must face the problem of a casting that cannot be brought into an acceptable fit in the mouth. Often it will not be possible to determine the cause of the poor fit. The fit of the frame on the master cast will often show that the laboratory phase of construction has produced a frame that fits the cast in an acceptable manner. If this is true, one can only conclude that the error was not in the laboratory. The clinician must then review the procedures for making the master impression. I feel that the inaccurate master cast can most often be traced to patient movement during the setting of the alginate gel or to separation of the alginate from the tray during removal of the impression. If one assumes that the alginate was prepackaged and mixed for the recommended length of time and that a careful double-pour technique was used to create the master cast, there really is no other place to look.

The removable partial denture framework is not an easy casting to make with precision. The geometry of the frame and the variations that can occur just from differences in expansion based on placement in the casting ring make the framework far more complex than in the casting of a crown. One could well expect to find 1 out of 8 or 10 castings unacceptable if one's standards of acceptance are high. It only makes sense to reward the excellent technician if one is fortunate enough to find one.

7

Completion of the Partial Denture

Once the framework has been properly fitted and found to be acceptable, the remaining steps in the construction of the advanced RPD are not all that different from the standard RPD. Certainly, attention to detail in the coloring of the denture base and the creation of metal occlusal surfaces merit our attention. The insertion of the RPD should go smoothly if the level of quality has been maintained throughout. It is clearly in the maintenance of the partial where the long-term success of the treatment will be determined.

Jaw Relation Records

Jaw relation records are normally made only after the framework has been fitted to the mouth and brought into the desired occlusal relationship with the opposing arch. Remember, if the master cast can be related to the opposing cast by simply placing the casts in occlusion with wear facets for reference, this will always be the method of choice. Only when this stable relationship is not obtainable should a record be made. The most positive recordings are made in a material that is truly plastic for the recording and then rapidly sets to a hard surface. Registration materials using zinc oxide with eugenol (ZnOe) as a base are most often used. Bosworth's Super Bite or Blue Mousse by Parkell are excellent examples of this type of material. They require a base of hard wax, trimmed to be 2 to 3 mm out of occlusion, as a platform for the actual recording. The setting time can generally be decreased by adding a small amount of water or alcohol to the mix. Once set, these materials can be trimmed with a sharp knife so that only the tips of the opposing cusps are visible (Fig 7-1). Since the opposing cusp tips are more likely to have been accurately reproduced in the opposing cast than in the full occlusal surface, the record should be easily verified when using this technique. The hard wax base should not contact the soft tissue in a Class III situation. Only on terminally edentulous areas is it necessary to obtain some support from the soft tissue.

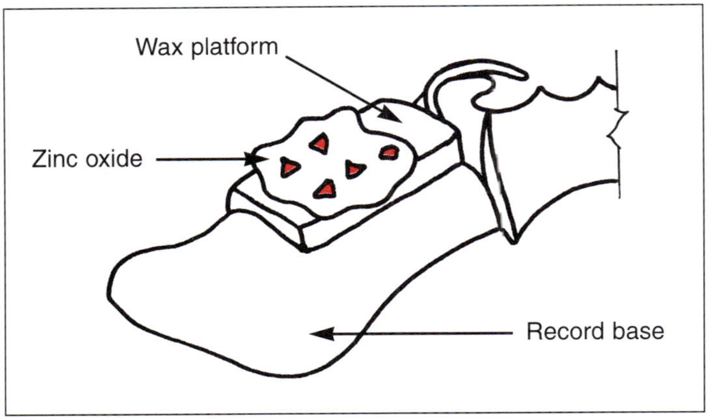

Fig 7-1 Zinc oxide record with only opposing cusp tips recorded.

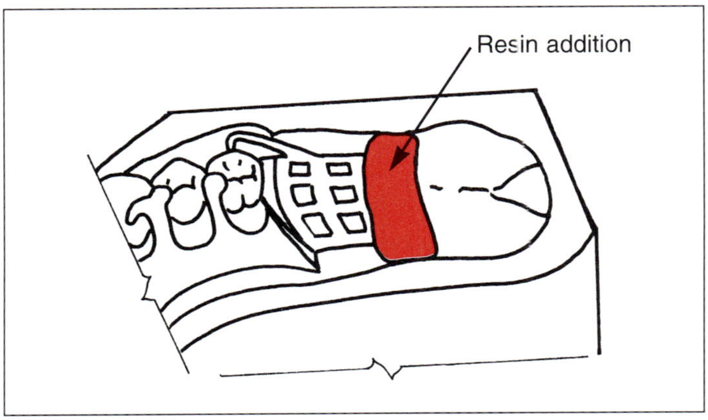

Fig 7-2 Autopolymerizing resin support for record added to posterior meshwork.

Since the ZnOe pastes are truly plastic for a short time after mixing, the record could theoretically be made without any posterior support. A compromise between no support and a full tissue base coverage can be made by placing an island of autopolymerizing resin under the place where the tissue stop is (or was) located, after the cast has been coated with a separating agent (Fig 7-2). This will reestablish the tissue stop support of the distal extension framework as well as serve as a base for the strip of hard wax that supports the recording material.

There is little evidence to support the making of a face-bow record for the removable partial denture case with natural teeth in the opposing arch. Only when the opposing arch is a complete denture could an argument be made for the use of an ear-bow or other arbitrary mounting. The great majority of removable partial dentures sent to a commercial laboratory for set-up and processing will use a plane line articulator. Protrusive records to set condylar inclination are also of little use because the plane line articulator is not adjustable.

Jaw relation records for a removable partial denture opposed by a complete denture require a much more involved technique. These records are most often made as a part of a separate appointment during which anterior teeth will be positioned and the basic records taken. When an altered

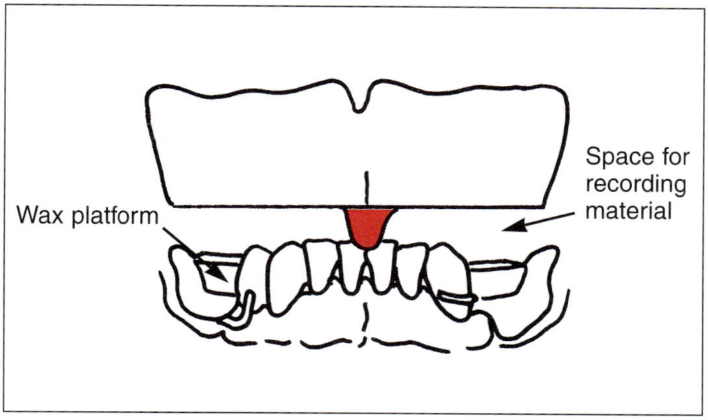

Fig 7-3 Use of cone in wax or compound to establish occluding vertical dimension.

cast impression is involved, that impression must be made before the jaw relation appointment. On occasion, a suitable record can be made in conjunction with the altered cast impression as described earlier.

The relationship sought for the CD/RPD situation is centric relation, not centric occlusion as with the other partial denture types. Either a processed denture base for the opposing arch or one made with a combination of plasticized resin (Lynal or similar material) and fast-setting orthodontic resin needs to be available for the centric relation record. The record must capture centric jaw relation, a posterior, unstrained, patient-assumed position at a vertical dimension of occlusion that allows the establishment of an esthetically pleasing face height, adequate speaking space, and some interocclusal space at rest, much the same as is required for a complete denture.

The first step is to establish the vertical dimension of occlusion. A quick and dependable method for finding and capturing this position of mandible to maxilla involves first establishing a length of wax rim that will extend short of the length of the relaxed upper lip by 2 to 3 mm. The patient is instructed to close to first contact and the face height is evaluated. The patient must appear obviously overclosed at this time. This does not in any way simulate the vertical position of the anterior teeth, as tooth placement is independent of the jaw relation record. A cone of wax or compound, warmed in a compound heater, is added to the wax rim in the midline of the maxilla. This cone is directed to contact the incisal edge of one of the mandibular anterior teeth, usually a central incisor (Fig 7-3). When no natural anterior teeth are present in the lower arch, a denture tooth (incisor) is arbitrarily placed onto the resin retention in the central incisor area. The cone is long enough to ensure that the vertical dimension of occlusion is exceeded at first contact. The patient is instructed to close, in centric relation, into the cone until the clinician tells the patient to stop—when the face looks neither overopened or overclosed. The clinician then evaluates the esthetic face height and repeats the procedure as necessary. The cone is allowed to harden to preserve the tentative vertical dimension record. After the cone has hardened so that it will not distort, any excess material can be removed so that only the incisal edge of the tooth remains in the record.

The contact of the cone and the incisor tooth will normally be visible to the clinician so that the speaking space can be evaluated. The amount of space seen when sibilant sounds are spoken will usually give an indication that the necessary "speaking space" has been created. Unfortunately, speech is not a good measure until all the teeth are present in the dentures of both arches and the patient has had time to adapt to the new contours. The clinician can, however, easily evaluate the interocclusal space at rest by looking at the relationship of the tip of the cone and the opposing tooth, even if the lips have to be slightly parted by hand to gain a line of sight. One could expect to see anywhere from 1.5 to 6 or 7 mm of space at rest, with the Class III patient having the least and the Class II the most. Finding the ideal vertical dimension at rest requires the balancing of these different factors. Since it is quite clear that there is no exact vertical dimension of occlusion, the clinician need only find an esthetic and comfortable dimension and then verify that position later with the trial set-up.

The cone, as it contacts the mandibular incisor, will also serve as a visual indicator of centric relation for the actual recording. To make the record as positive and as foolproof as possible for others to mount casts into the articulator, one can place a molar denture tooth on each side of the maxillary rim in the area of the first and second molars (Fig 7-4). The cusps of these denture teeth will imprint on the recording material with a minimum of pressure and leave precise indentations so that, with the cone as the third point of reference, a positive record can be easily verified visually, both in the mouth and when mounting the master casts. Instead of using a new denture tooth for this purpose, unused teeth, always available in the office, can be cut in half horizontally so that no interference will occur when placing the occlusal portion onto the maxillary rim. This method is always superior to cutting grooves in the rim and expecting the recording material to flow up into the grooves.

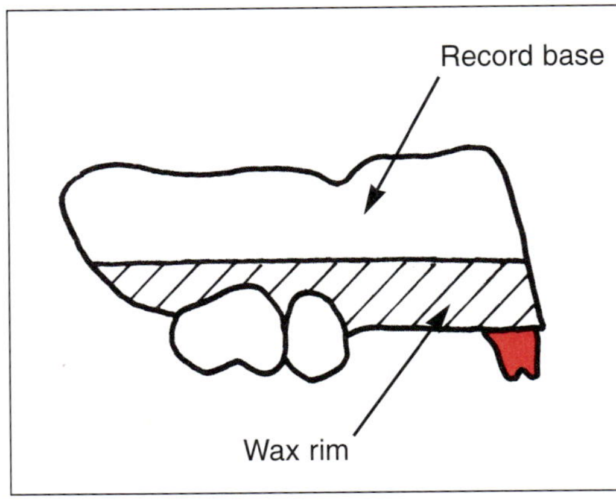

Fig 7-4 Lateral view of maxillary record base with cone and posterior denture teeth.

Placement of Denture Teeth

The occlusion desired for RPD situations where the opposing arch contains natural teeth restored in any manner is one of contact in centric occlusion only. Disclusion, both in lateral movements and in protrusion, should not occur on the denture teeth, if at all possible. When denture teeth must be involved in disclusion, as when a canine is replaced, some form of metal cov-

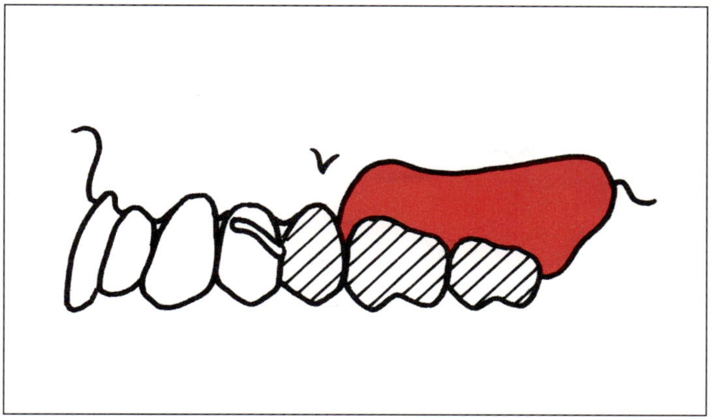

Fig 7-5 Denture flange begins distal to the most anterior tooth.

erage on the denture tooth must be considered to eliminate the rapid wear that can be expected with resin against porcelain, natural teeth, or restorative materials.

For those situations in which the opposing dentition is a complete denture, the partial denture occlusion should be similar to that of standard complete dentures—some form of working and balancing contacts over a range of 1 to 1.5 mm from the centric position. Protrusive contacts are often not possible to obtain without drastically altering the vertical and horizontal overlaps of the anterior teeth, which will most likely be unacceptable esthetically.

Before placing the first denture teeth onto the partial framework, consideration must be given to the contour of the resin flange. Since severe resorption of the residual ridge is unlikely to occur immediately adjacent to an abutment tooth, the first denture tooth will be much more likely to appear natural if it is butted to the ridge and the flange is begun in the interproximal area between the first and second tooth (Fig 7-5). A denture tooth of sufficient occlusogingival length must be chosen to allow a natural transition between it and the abutment tooth. Often this implies a tooth with a well-formed and colored root surface (as is found on the Ivoclar posterior tooth, for example). Should the abutment tooth be clasped with a circumferential clasp, the denture tooth will have to be carefully contoured to create space for the clasp to exit without causing an esthetically unacceptable display of base material. Should too much of the denture tooth be removed for placement, the resulting unnatural denture base can be removed with a cavity preparation in the resin and a microfilled composite placed to simulate a proximal restoration after processing and finishing the partial denture (Fig 7-6).

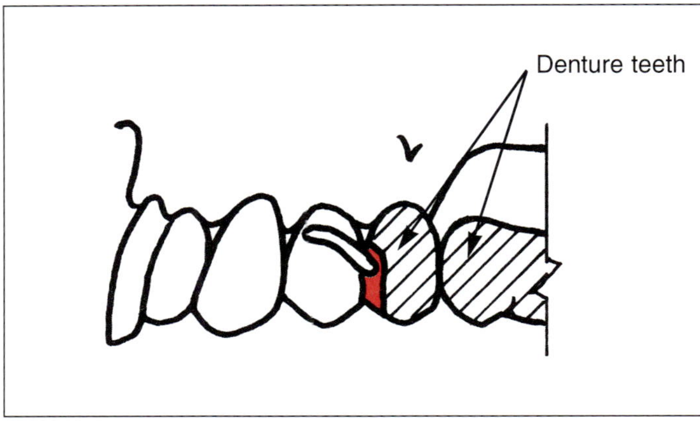

Fig 7-6 Use of composite restoration to disguise clasp exit.

With the CD/RPD, it is not always possible to position the denture tooth in the ideal position that would be used in a CD/CD situation. Remaining natural teeth will often require the use of diastemas or crowding of the denture teeth to properly interdigitate with the opposing complete denture. The mesial aspect of the first denture tooth should not be compromised, since any extra space here will fill with base resin and be esthetically unacceptable, especially if the abutment tooth has a circumferential clasp. (This will occur primarily when that tooth is the prime abutment for a Class I or II situation, because anterior clasping will not normally occur on the Class III partial.)

The same mesiodistal considerations mentioned above can be expected to occur when the partial denture is opposed by natural teeth, with or without a partial denture. In addition, the contour of the occlusal surface of the denture tooth will often not harmonize with the occlusal surface of the natural tooth. To obtain good esthetics with maximum centric contact, the denture tooth may need to be placed in hyperocclusion and then ground into a solid centric contact. When this need arises, the clinician must verify that a denture tooth of the same dimensions as the natural tooth has been selected. The manufacturer's recommended mold, as taken from the mold guide of any anterior tooth, cannot be used, as it will always be too small to allow optimum occlusal contact. Instead, the choice of the posterior tooth mold will be made only on the basis of the mesiodistal and buccolingual dimensions of the opposing natural tooth. In the same manner, the choice of cusp height is based on the contours of the opposing teeth.

In most instances, a 1-mm hyperocclusion that is adjusted into contact will be satisfactory. The occlusal surface of the adjusted tooth must be recontoured to recreate the occlusal anatomy, usually by reestablishing the grooves and fossae with an inverted cone bur. Denture teeth should be positioned and ground into suitable occlusal contact one at a time instead of setting all the teeth into hyperocclusion at once, since some teeth will require a greater or lesser degree of hyperocclusion than others.

As the positioning of the teeth proceeds posteriorly (or anteriorly in the case of the Class IV), the creation of small, randomized diastemas will usually result in a lifelike appearance of any teeth that are visible. Likewise, if anterior teeth are included, they will need to be selected, and decisions made as to diastemas or crowding, on the basis of the dimension of the edentulous area. Because anterior diastemas are unlikely to occur in one arch only, the most common placement will be in an area with some level of crowding. Remember, it is very unlikely that any patient requiring anterior tooth replacement in the mandible would have perfectly straight incisors unless the patient is very young or has a tooth-arch discrepancy that would indicate the need for diastemas. Obviously, the patient can be expected to remember the presence of diastemas but may not recall the crowding.

Second molars would be placed in the mandibular partial denture only when the opposing arch contains second molars that have the potential for continued eruption or the opposing arch is a complete denture and the patient is severely Class III. In the maxillary arch the second molar may be partially visible and therefore should be replaced.

For the removable partial denture opposed by a complete denture (almost always CD/RPD), some decision on the occlusal scheme of the combined prosthesis must be made. There is no evidence that one form of occlusal arrangement is superior to any other, but for esthetic reasons some form of cusped tooth is usually indicated because a flat tooth may be difficult to harmonize with the remaining natural teeth. Perhaps the lingualized arrangement is the most adaptable.

Final waxing and waxing for try-in, should that be indicated, must be identical, except that the final waxing includes sealing the perpheries. Unfortunately, waxing for try-in is often done in a casual manner, which does not allow the clinician to fully evaluate the final form and esthetics of the denture. The wax-up must always be evaluated off the cast to ensure that adequate thickness of base material will be available after finishing and polishing. Any areas of potential sore spots, as might be found adjacent to a sharp mylohyoid ridge, should be overwaxed and then recontoured in the final resin once any problems of pressure spots have been eliminated. Any flange area for which tinting of the denture base material is planned must be waxed to exacting contours, since the tinting will be superficial and easily altered by recontouring. Those flange margins that will be visible must be waxed to a very thin margin and should be slightly curved as they pass vertically, since a straight line will tend to be more visible than a margin that flows with the contours of the tissues. As a final step in the waxing of the denture base, all traces of wax must be removed from the exposed denture teeth. This is normally done with a sharp carving instrument, such as a Walls carver. Further use of the flame will result in a flash of wax, so it should be avoided. The object of this final waxing is to create a surface that will require no finishing, only a light polishing, since any finishing operation will remove some of the outer surface of the tooth and the tinted denture base.

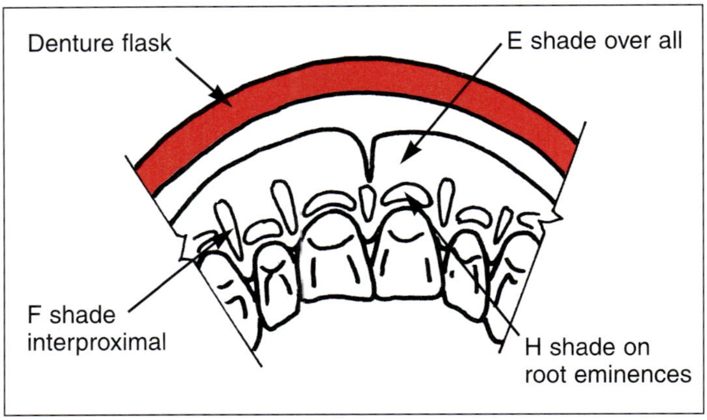

Fig 7-7 Denture base tinting guide for fair-skinned patient (Dr Pound).

Flasking, Tinting, and Packing

The laboratory procedures of flasking and packing the removable partial denture are more complex than those of the complete denture and, except for the tinting of the denture base, are not highly technique sensitive. Since there may often be many small areas of isolated base resin, a split packing of the flask is used. The technique of split packing implies that a sheet of cellophane, with resin on both sides, is kept between the halves of the flask up to the final closure of the denture flasks. This procedure ensures that the resin will not pull out of the interproximal areas or from around clasp arms during trial packing. At the final closure, the cellophane is removed and the two resin surfaces are moistened with monomer to ensure a complete bond.

The tinting of the flange is one of the techniques that makes the difference between a standard denture and a state-of-the-art prosthesis. As part of the tinting of the denture base, consideration must be given to opaquing the casting in areas where the grayness of the metal may show through thin sections of the flange. Resins associated with the 4-META bonding agents can be used to bond on a thin layer of opaque that is suitably colored, but experimentation with coloration will be required between clinician and technician.

Certainly, tinting to accurately match the patient's gingival color is a matter of art rather than science and, unfortunately, something that cannot be done at the chair. Superficial tints are available but they are only temporary in nature. Definitive tinting requires that the tinted resins (available from Kay-See Dental Mfg Co, Kansas City, MO, for Dr Earl Pound's "sift in" technique) be placed in the flask and blended from the outside inward before the regular base material is added (Fig 7-7). The clinician interested in developing this aspect for the "advanced" partial denture must create a series of shade tabs in conjunction with the dental laboratory that will process the resin. The Kay-See kit contains five vials of colored polymer that range from a very light pink, used to tint

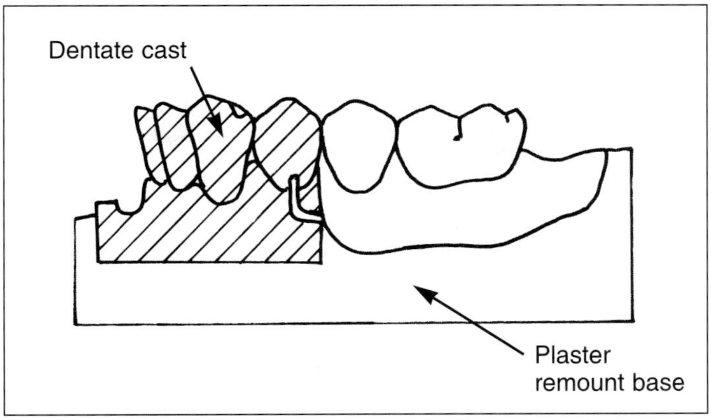

Fig 7-8 Remount cast for RPD.

areas of firmly attached tissue over the necks of teeth, to a dark, heavily pigmented color that is compatible with darker tinting patterns. The kit also contains red flocking that can be placed in the areas of unattached gingiva to simulate blood vessels. The short flocking that is commonly found in denture base materials does not look natural, especially when it appears in the marginal gingiva in a random pattern, as can be expected with standard packing techniques. This type of flocking does, however, add color to otherwise partially translucent material. When the tints are placed in the outer surface of the base and backed up with the standard resin, the end result can be indistinguishable from natural tissue. Since a natural appearance of the visible denture base is critical to ideal esthetics, mastery of the tinting process is an essential component of an advanced level of prosthodontic care. The instructions that come with the tinting kit provide sufficient guidance for choosing the appropriate colors but do not cover the fine points of their application.

Because the denture base adjacent to the denture teeth has been carefully waxed to the desired contour, the final finishing of the finished denture base should require only the removal of the flash from the packing and the possible slight reshaping and polishing of the denture borders. Finishing and polishing of the junction of the denture tooth and the base should be kept to a minimum for the most esthetically pleasing result.

Should the partial denture be Class I or II and opposed by a complete denture, a remount cast must be made for the finished prosthesis. Occasionally, the dentate portion of the master cast can be salvaged in deflasking but, more often than not, the cast is destroyed in the process. A second pour of the dentate portion of the final impression is perfectly adequate for the remount cast. The finished partial is placed on the dentate portion, and a plaster base is added to support the distal extensions (Fig 7-8). Any undercuts present in the denture bases must be blocked out before pouring the plaster base.

Insertion

Because of the care taken to make the altered cast impression, there should be little adjustment of the denture base at insertion. Flanges of tooth-borne segments should be short of any undercut areas. Pressure-indicator paste will identify areas of possible subsequent sore spots, but it is important to remember that the correlation of a visible spot in the pressure paste and a subsequent area of soreness is not 100%. Therefore, some thought must be given before removing denture base material. The most common areas that require adjustment are areas of tissue undercuts, below the height of contour, normally found adjacent to the terminal abutments (Fig 7-9). The guiding planes will dictate the path of insertion. The resin in these usually minor undercuts must be relieved even if the undercuts do not initially hinder the full seating of the denture. The soft tissue in these areas is usually quite thin over the bone and tightly bound. To avoid traumatizing these tissues, the partial denture should never be fully seated at first. Rather, pressure-indicating paste is painted on the resin, and the partial is seated until the first slight resistance is felt or the patient feels pressure. The partial is removed and adjusted, and this careful procedure is repeated until the partial fully seats without any feeling of pressure or rubbing expressed by the patient. By starting the flange of the denture base distal to the first denture tooth as was described earlier, some of these problems can be eliminated.

Retentive clasp arms may have been distorted in the deflasking process and may require adjustment at insertion. Rather than trying to overadapt the clasps, the patient is better served by leaving the partial on the loose side with the explanation that the initial goal is to have the partial only minimally retentive. Since all prosthodontic patients will have at least one postinsertion visit within the first few days, further adjustment of the clasps can be done at that time if the patient finds the initial retention inadequate. Most patients will understand that having the partial too rigidly attached to the remaining teeth is not desirable in the long run.

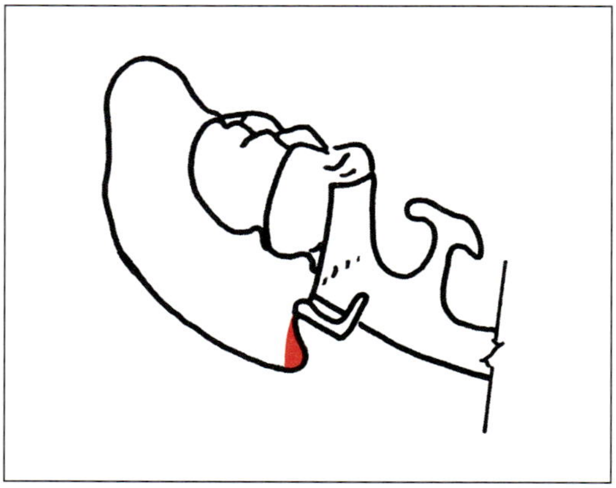

Fig 7-9 Critical undercut area generally requiring adjustment before seating the RPD.

Occlusal adjustments are almost always required at the insertion appointment. This should be looked on as fortuitous because the absence of prematurities often means infraocclusion, which can only be corrected by the addition of metal occlusals. The patient should not be released if the natural teeth are not back in contact with the opposing occlusion, unless some type of overall onlay casting has been deliberately selected to increase occluding vertical dimension. If the patient has a partial denture in both arches, the partials should be adjusted one at a time to natural tooth contacts before attempting to place

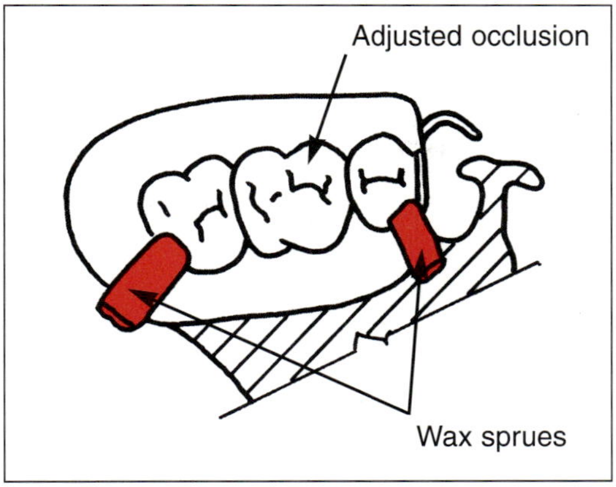

Fig 7-10 Sprue leads attached to build metal occlusal surfaces.

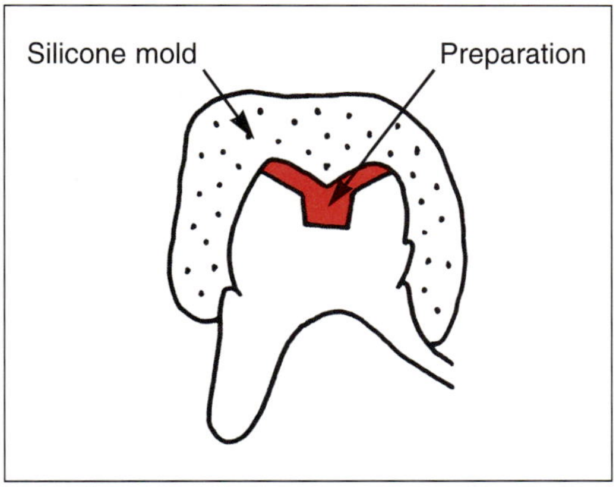

Fig 7-11 Silicone mold to duplicate occlusal surfaces.

both partials in the mouth for final adjustment. Any easily visible natural tooth contact can be chosen as a witness mark to be sure that natural tooth contact occurs, both in centric occlusion and in excursive movements.

A postinsertion visit within 3 days of the insertion appointment is essential to complete the insertion procedure. If all aspects of construction have been accomplished with care, there is seldom need for any additional postinsertion appointments. The patient can be placed on a well-defined recall program at this point, realizing that only through regular recall and reevaluation can the full life of the partial denture be assured.

Metal Occlusal Surfaces

When the removable partial denture is opposed by natural teeth or fixed restorations, consideration must be given to protecting the occlusal surfaces from the inevitable wear that occurs. There are many techniques for fabricating metal occlusions. Perhaps the most dependable method is to allow the patient to wear the new partial denture for a month or so to be certain that the chosen occlusal scheme is appropriate for that situation. At that point, the patient returns and the partial is placed back on the remount cast, if one has been made for adjustment at insertion. Sprue leads of 6-gauge round wax (or similar wax forms) are added to the occlusal table, one at the most posterior cusp and one at the most anterior (Fig 7-10). Then a silicone mold is made of the occlusal surfaces of the denture teeth to include the sprue leads. Using a resin finishing bur, the occlusal surfaces of the denture teeth are reduced by a uniform 1 mm, including the grooves. A 3-mm-deep central groove is cut into the teeth (and, in some instances, extends into the denture base material). This groove should be wide enough to occupy a third of the buccolingual width of the teeth (Fig 7-11).

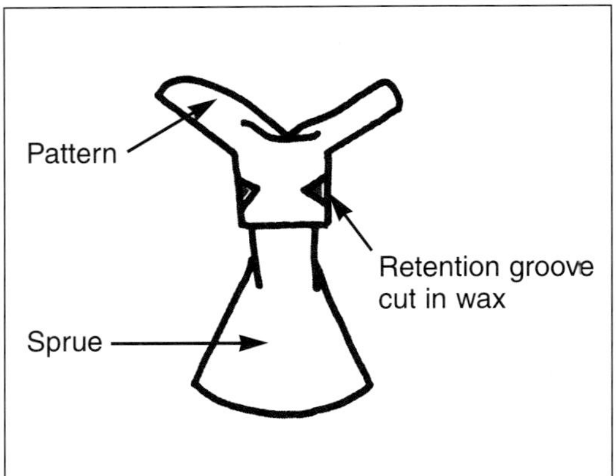

Fig 7-12 Sprued wax pattern with retention grooves.

The occlusal surfaces of the denture teeth and groove are lubricated with a separating material, and the silicone mold(s) are replaced on the partial. Molten inlay wax is injected, using an eye dropper, into one of the sprue leads until wax is seen coming out the opposite sprue. When the wax has cooled, the silicone molds are removed and any voids or defects are corrected with additional wax. In partials for which no remount cast was made, the wax contacts can be verified in the mouth. When the desired occlusal contacts are obtained, the wax occlusal block is teased from the denture and sprued from the underside of the central groove with sufficient sprue leads to assure a complete casting. Before investing the wax patterns, a retentive groove is cut into the bulk of wax that extends into the central groove (Fig 7-12). The purpose of this groove is to ensure physical retention of the casting in the denture base. A 4 META–type bonding agent can be applied to the casting as an additional retentive measure. The partial denture is cleansed and reinserted, and the patient is dismissed. Since it will take only a day or two to invest, cast, and finish the casting, the patient can use the partial in a normal fashion even if mastication is somewhat compromised.

When the castings have been finished, the patient returns and the partial is placed on the remount cast (if one exists) to complete the process. The tooth-colored resin that will be used to join the casting to the teeth will be viscous, so additional space for the resin will need to be created by removing a small amount of tooth substance overall. The casting is tried into the preparation and if the occlusal contacts are satisfactory, tooth-colored resin of the appropriate shade is mixed and placed in the groove, on the other prepared surfaces, and in the retentive groove on the casting. The casting is forced to place by closing the articulator to the original occlusal vertical dimension. Excess tooth-colored resin is removed and then a stout rubber band is placed around the articulator to hold the casts in occlusion while the articulator is placed in the pressure pot. After finishing and polishing, the metal occlusal surfaces can be expected to add considerable life to the removable partial denture. The only potential problem with this procedure is that there will be microleakage at the metal-resin interface that will, in time, leave a dark line in the resin. By using a bonding agent, this line can be eliminated or greatly reduced.

Depending on the opposing occlusion, the metal occlusal surfaces need not cover the entire occlusal surface of the denture teeth. They may, in fact, take the form of large Class I restorations. When the opposing occlusion is a complete denture, the lingual cusps of the posterior teeth can be made in metal using the same technique. A lingualized occlusion that virtually eliminates occlusal wear for the expected life of the dentures can be created for the patient.

Long-Term Maintenance

Long-term maintenance of a partial denture constructed to the highest standards, as described in this book, will be minimal and limited to the occasional readjustment of retentive clasp arms and precision attachments. Resilient attachments can be expected to need replacement on an annual basis. Relines of distal extension bases and areas of recent extraction will be required when indicated. An evaluation of the fit of the resin denture base must be a part of the annual recall appointment.

Of far greater importance in the recall and maintenance phase of treatment is the continued management of both the periodontal and restorative components. Excellent studies indicate that the life expectancy of a removable partial denture can be increased toward 20 years if the supporting structures can be maintained. Remember, the partial denture patient has already demonstrated some degree of inability to manage his/her own disease process, with the exception of traumatic and congenital needs for care. In the first year after insertion, the patient should be seen at either 3 or 6 months to evaluate the response of the tissues to the partial denture. An essential part of this recall is the evaluation of the patient's ability to clean not only the remaining teeth, but the partial denture as well. The use of a solution of vegetable dye to stain the partial will generally indicate those areas where plaque remains. Often, the clinician will find that the patient has lost the denture brush that is normally provided at the insertion appointment and is trying to clean the partial with a standard toothbrush that may not have bristles of sufficient length to get into all areas. The standard of clinical care has not been met until patients have proven their ability to keep the partial free from accumulations of plaque.

8

Repairs, Additions, and Relines

Many of the necessary repairs and additions to a removable partial denture will, by necessity, be made in the dental laboratory. It is incumbent on the clinician, however, to be knowledgeable in the area of framework repairs and to fully understand the clinical requirements necessary to prepare the prosthesis for the laboratory repair.

Pick-up Impressions

The clinician will be responsible for relating the partial to the mouth and for capturing this relationship in the pick-up impression, regardless of the type of repair or addition. To be certain that the partial denture is fully seated during the impression, the clinician will often be required to hold the partial in position while the impression is being made. This requirement necessitates a sectional impression. Fortunately, repairs are almost always confined to one specific area of the denture, so that a pick-up impression that covers only the quadrant in question will allow the partial to be held firmly in position. In some instances, an assistant will be required to seat the tray while the clinician maintains the components in position. When a pick-up impression, almost always made in irreversible hydrocolloid, is fully set, every attempt should be made to remove both the impression and the partial together. Should the alginate separate from the partial, the clinician must be certain that the prosthesis has been fully reseated in the impression. This will sometimes require small amounts of impression material, which may have been bent under the partial during reinsertion, to be cut from the impression before the pouring of the repair cast.

When pouring the repair cast, only the portion of the arch that relates to the actual repair need be reproduced on the cast. As long as there is sufficient cast structure to ensure that the technician can remove and replace the segment(s) accurately, there is no advantage to having a larger cast. In fact, it is often easier to work with a partial cast, since seating the repair on and off the cast is facilitated and the possibility of cast fracture reduced.

Resin Repairs

The need to repair only a resin portion of the properly constructed removable partial denture is usually related to an accident in which the patient has dropped the partial and some part of the denture base fractured. When the broken part is available, it can usually be repositioned exactly based on the fracture line. It is then a simple matter to submit the denture and the fractured resin to the laboratory for repair. Occasionally, the patient will attempt to repair the fracture using the dreaded Super Glue. Once this material has been placed on the resin, accurate repositioning of the two segments is usually impossible. In this instance, the Super Glue is removed with an acrylic bur and the remainder of the denture base is prepared for a reline impression.

Approximately 1 mm of denture resin is removed from the entire tissue surface of the fractured denture base, and the missing or broken area is reformed using gray or green stick modeling compound. Once the borders of the defect have been corrected, 1 mm of compound is removed from the tissue side of the addition and a wash reline impression is made in the affected denture base. The wash impression can be made in any free-flowing impression material. The completed reline impression is submitted to the laboratory, a cast is poured against the impression, and the reline and repair are completed at the same time, either in a flask or a reline jig. By combining the repair with a reline, an accurate tissue surface is obtained regardless of the fracture site.

Another common repair situation is the fracture of an isolated denture tooth, almost always caused by inadequate framework design and construction. Since the cause of the fracture is in the framework, no successful, long-term repair can be made without either remaking the specific retentive component or using one of the modern resin-to-metal bonding agents (4-META). Since the cost of remaking and soldering on a proper retentive element approaches the cost of a new casting, the bonding agents offer an inexpensive and apparently dependable method of single tooth repair. The proper use of these bonding agents is technique-sensitive; the manufacturer's instructions must be followed to the letter.

Metal Repairs

The most common metal repairs are associated with fractured clasp arms. For the most part, these fractured clasps can be replaced with a wrought clasp. Embrasure clasps and clasps emerging from some single-tooth edentulous spaces are the exceptions to the rule and may not be reparable. Whenever possible, a fractured cast circumferential clasp, the most commonly used clasp, should be replaced with an infrabulge wire clasp, since the replacement clasp will be contained entirely in the resin of the denture base and not involve the occlusal surfaces (Fig 8-1). When infrabulge clasps are added as the repair clasp, the technician must be reminded that the approach arm of the clasp must not contact the gingiva if the partial can be expected to

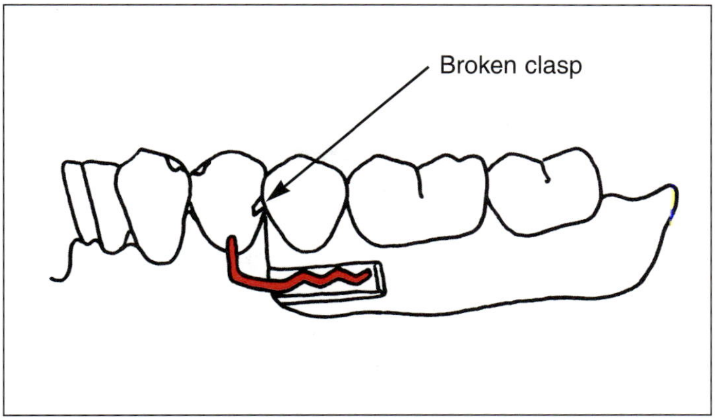

Fig 8-1 Replacement of a circumferential clasp with a wire I-bar.

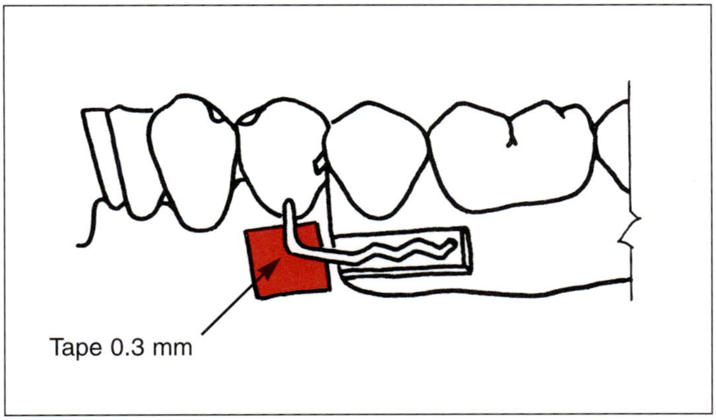

Fig 8-2 Adhesive tape square used to keep repair clasp off tissue.

rotate into the soft tissue, as it would if it were a Class I partial. Instead, the clasp should be positioned so that it is slightly away (0.2 to 0.3 mm) from the soft tissue (Fig 8-2).

Before making the pick-up impression, the cause of the clasp fracture, if known, should be evaluated. It may be that the clasp was poorly designed or constructed, that without some additional mouth preparation the situation cannot be improved, and that the repaired clasp will itself fracture in the future. This is most commonly seen in circumferential clasps where insufficient space for the clasp was created during mouth preparation and the clasp arm or shoulder was adjusted to allow full occlusal contact of the opposing teeth. The adjustment created a thin spot that became a point of stress concentration and resulted in the fracture. The thickness of the metal at the fracture site can be measured and, if it is less than 1.2 mm, additional mouth preparation must be accomplished before the impression. For similar reasons, other tooth contours are modified to the ideal form, line angles are rounded, and excessive undercuts are reduced as an essential component of the repair procedure.

After all indicated mouth preparation has been done, the pick-up impression is made. Again, the need to maintain the par-

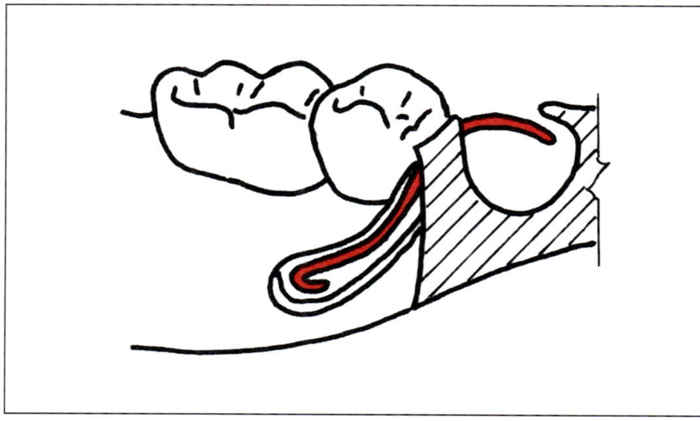

Fig 8-3 Lingual access for circumferential repair wire.

tial in its ideal relation to its supporting structures is essential, since the fractured clasp may eliminate the possibility that the partial will stay in place for a full-arch impression.

Rather than send the pick-up impression directly to the technician, the clinician must pour the cast and remove the denture after the stone has set so that the contours of the stone abutment tooth can be surveyed and the gauge and position of the replacement wire clasp determined and marked on the cast. The same standards of clasp construction discussed in earlier chapters apply to the repair clasp.

When the clasp in question does not have an adjacent acrylic flange of suitable proportions to allow the placement of an infrabulge clasp, the repair will require a circumferential clasp. This repair will involve the opening of the occlusal surface of the denture tooth adjacent to the repair so that the wire circumferential clasp can be brought transocclusally to be embedded in the lingual resin of the denture base (Fig 8-3). As a result of the preparation of the transocclusal groove, the occlusal surface of the denture tooth will need repair as well. To ensure that the repaired partial denture will have proper occlusal contact in this area, the opposing denture or cast of the opposing teeth should be sent to the lab with the repair cast so that the technician can restore the occlusal surface(s) involved.

The fractured embrasure clasp may be repaired by sectioning the lingual minor connector a few millimeters below the occlusal surface before making the pick-up impression so that the minor connector weld is not placed in an area of occlusal load (Fig 8-4). The laboratory can then block out the cast and duplicate, wax, and cast a replacement embrasure clasp. This clasp, when finished and polished, can be welded to the framework to complete the repair. Unfortunately, the cost of this type of repair is high and totally dependent on the weld for longevity. In most of these situations, it is advisable to remake the partial denture.

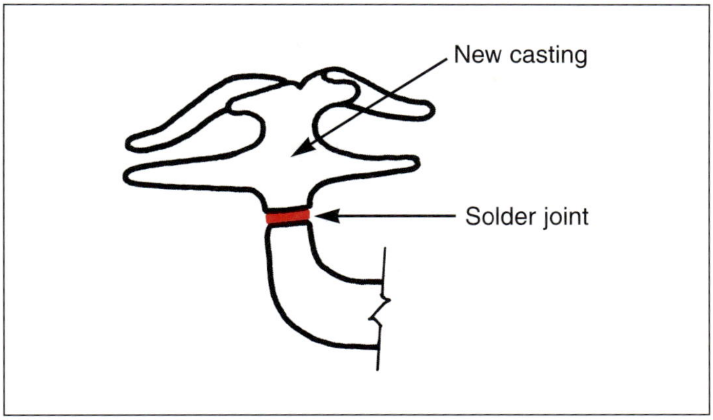

Fig 8-4 Repair of embrasure clasp.

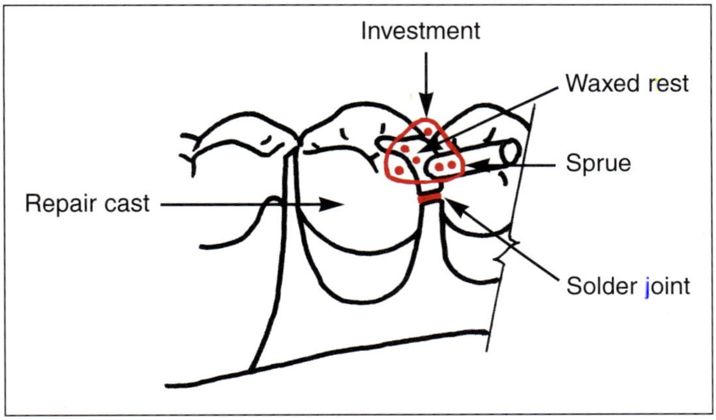

Fig 8-5 Replacement of broken occlusal rest.

The same procedure of sectioning the minor connector first is used for another common repair situation, that of the fractured occlusal rest. This type of fracture can almost always be blamed on inadequate mouth preparation that leaves a marginal ridge reduction of less than the 1.2 mm mentioned before. The technician can wax the replacement rest directly on the lubricated repair cast. The rest is sprued with a small round wax sprue lead, and a small amount of appropriate casting investment is painted on the wax (Fig 8-5). Once the investment has set, the entire assembly can be teased from the repair cast and added to some other partial denture framework casting for final investment and casting. The finished rest addition is polished and joined to the partial using 800 fine solder with a resistance brazing device as a heat source. This type of soldering is an art form and requires considerable skill and experience. High-quality laboratories with a reputation for removable partial denture frameworks can be expected to have such skills available to the clinician.

The addition of a denture tooth to the partial to replace a natural tooth lost to decay or periodontal disease is also a common repair situation, often one that could be considered a real emergency if the tooth happens to be an anterior. The tooth can be

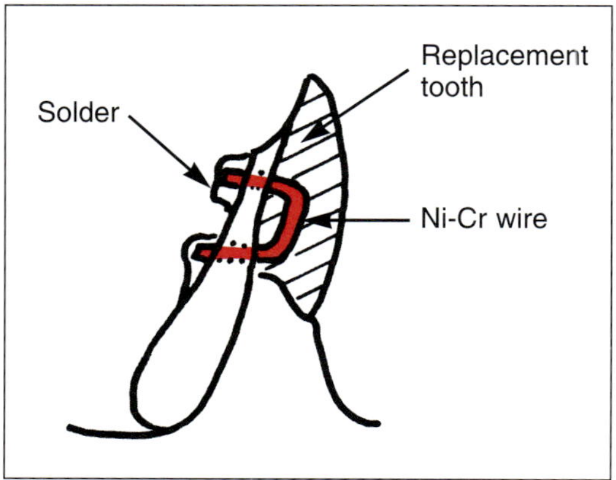

Fig 8-6 Addition of retention and denture tooth to lingual plate.

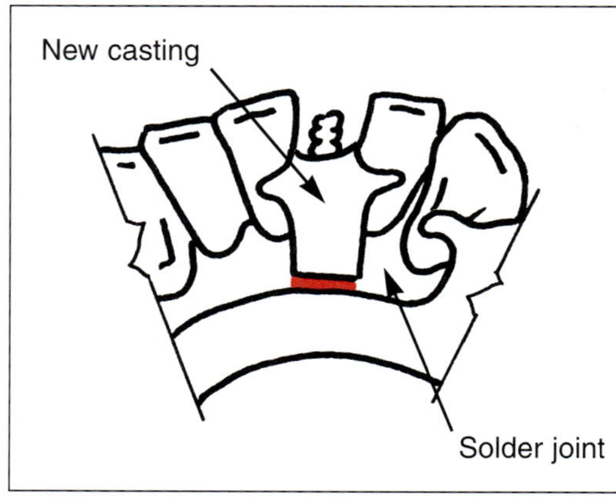

Fig 8-7 Addition of cast retention to lingual bar.

replaced as an addition after the natural tooth has been extracted and initial healing has taken place or, and this is often the preferred way, as an immediate replacement followed by the extraction. In either case, the existing framework must be capable of supporting the addition. As discussed earlier, one indication for a lingual plate is when the potential for tooth loss exists. When a lingual plate is present, the best results are obtained by drilling two small holes in the plate and soldering a small loop of wire, usually one of Ni, Cr, and Co, into the holes so that the loop is internal to the replacement denture tooth (Fig 8-6). This form of retention will be as strong as one that is part of a new partial framework. When no lingual plate exists and there is insufficient adjoining resin to retain the denture tooth, a cast addition is indicated (Fig 8-7). As in the replacement of the broken embrasure clasp, the cost of a quality repair may approach that of a new casting. Again, and on a temporary basis, the 4-META bonding agents can be used to add a tooth to the metal framework.

Fractures of major connectors can be repaired by using 800 fine solder and the resistance brazing device. Obviously, the mandibular bar will be the easiest major connector to weld, since it offers easy access over a limited distance. Maxillary major connector repairs are seldom worth the effort. The need for a major connector repair results more often from distortion rather than from outright fracture of the metal. The patient who drops a partial and then steps on it can expect it not to fit all that well from then on. In an emergency situation, the major connector can be separated with a thin disk at the point of the perceived bend; if both segments fit the mouth in an acceptable manner, it is worth making the pick-up impression and sending the case off to the laboratory for welding. Beyond this, major connector repair is not practical.

Restorations Under Existing RPDs

It is not uncommon for abutment teeth to require some form of restoration during the life of the partial denture. The two- or three-surface alloy restoration that fractures at the isthmus is difficult to place under an existing partial and maintain positive contact with the rest. In these instances, the tooth usually requires repreparation of the box form to widen, or deepen, or some combination of the two, to ensure that an adequate bulk of amalgam is present. These restorations may also be made in composite if the clinician is comfortable with its use in the posterior. Since the composite filling can be layered into the cavity, the final contact with the rest or other components of the partial can be made after the removal of the rubber dam and matrix. Light activation of the composite is usually possible in a two-stage process where the material is first activated with the partial in place. This will usually set the material sufficiently to allow removal of the partial denture without distorting the restoration. Additional light curing with the partial out of the mouth completes the restoration.

For those situations in which a complete composite restoration is not indicated, a combination of alloy and composite can be used to support an occlusal rest. After the additional mouth preparation, the alloy is packed in the usual manner and then a dovetailed box in the area of the rest is formed (Fig 8-8). Chemically curing composite is placed in the box, and the partial is fully seated in the mouth until completely cured. This combination of restorative materials will allow the creation of a positive rest seat contact. Some form of microfilled resin is indicated in these repair situations rather than any of the heavily filled materials.

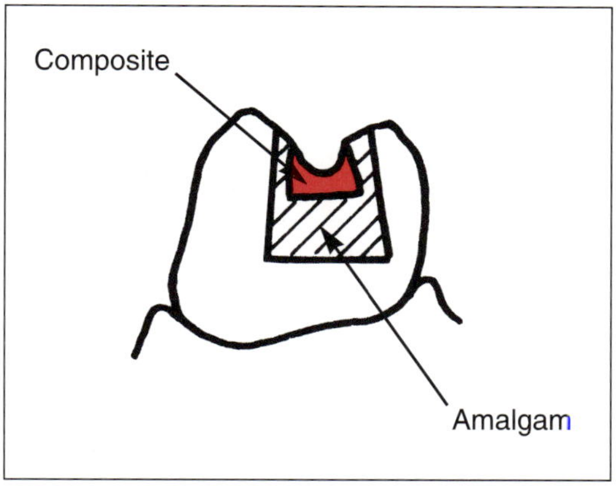

Fig 8-8 Composite and amalgam combination to retrofit rest.

Crowns Under Existing RPDs

In many situations, restoration of the tooth with amalgam or composite will not be adequate to support the partial or to properly restore the tooth. Some type of veneered or all-metal crown will be needed. Constructing a crown under an existing partial denture is not an easy task and, if it is not done to perfection, the partial will not seat passively on the tooth after cementation of the crown.

It is essential that sufficient tooth structure be left to allow for both retention and resistance forms, since the potential loading of the abutment tooth can be expected to be greater than for an uninvolved tooth. If inadequate tooth structure remains, then consideration should be given to either surgical crown lengthening or orthodontic extrusion. Only as a last resort should endodontic treatment with post and core be considered, since the failure rate for this approach with partial denture abutments is high.

In almost all these repair situations, the tooth will be prepared for a full crown. The clinician must verify that sufficient tooth structure has been removed to allow a minimum of 0.5 mm of metal on the axial walls and up to 2.0 mm on the occlusal surface if an occlusal rest is involved.

As in other repair situations, the impression must be made with the partial denture in its proper relationship to the supporting abutment teeth. This requires a sectional impression with the clinician holding the partial in position while the assistant seats the sectional tray. The actual impression is made by removing the retraction cord and injecting the low-viscosity impression material of choice completely around the margin of the preparation. A small amount of impression material can be injected onto the remainder of the prepared tooth. An excess of material might restrict the full seating of the partial.

The partial denture is seated in the mouth, and additional material is syringed onto the prepared tooth and into the space between the tooth and the partial. Once the space is filled with the low-viscosity material, the sectional tray can be seated. This tray must extend on either side of the repair area so that there will be sufficient impression material to lock the partial into the impression. The impression and the partial must be removed at one time because the chance of being able to accurately reposition the partial into the impression is unlikely. The master cast is then poured, either by the clinician if the partial is to be returned to the patient, or by the technician if the partial is to be kept in the laboratory for the construction of the crown. When pouring the master cast, it is critical that the stone be poured directly against all parts of the partial denture with the exception of clasp arms, precision attachments, and undercuts in the resin areas. This will allow a positive seating of the casting during the construction of the repair crown.

If the patient can do without the partial denture for the time that it takes to complete the repair, then the technician need only marginate the die and wax the crown to fit the framework. This is usually done by first waxing a thin coping to the margins. The casting is then seated on the cast, and molten wax is flowed in the space between the coping and the casting, using a glass eyedropper that has been warmed in the flame to prevent the wax from cooling too quickly.

The most difficult part of the repair is waxing the area where the clasp, should there be one, will lie. Not only will the wax need to flow against the internal area of the clasp arm, but a retentive contour will have to be built into the wax-up. The undercut formed from this contour will have to relate to the path of insertion and provide the required 0.010-inch dimension for the terminal third of the clasp arm. If the crown is to have a porcelain veneer, the task becomes even more difficult, since the porcelain must be overbuilt originally. As a result, the frame cannot be removed from the crown without fracturing off the dry porcelain.

The solution to these problems is to sacrifice the retentive clasp arm and make the facial contour to ideal dimensions. After the porcelain veneering is complete, with appropriate undercut in place, a repair clasp is added to the partial using the techniques previously described. The resulting repair crown will have an ideal form and will often be an improvement, both functionally and esthetically, over the original abutment tooth.

Should the patient require the use of the partial denture during the repair period, the clinician will need to pour and recover the final impression and construct a temporary restoration in the shape of the original tooth form. A vacuum form made from a diagnostic cast before mouth preparation can be used to make the temporary. Another technique uses a putty matrix that is made of the tooth before preparation. Missing tooth structure can be restored with soft wax before the matrix is adapted to the tooth. After preparation, the matrix is filled with tooth-colored resin and seated on the preparation. Unfortunately, some adjustment of the temporary is almost always required to seat the partial denture. Areas of premature contact are best identified using the Mylar-based articulating ribbon placed inside the partial contours when the frame is seated onto the temporary crown. Points of heavy contact show up easily and are adjusted.

The patient is allowed to wear the partial denture but is asked to return once the die has been trimmed and a wax coping has been dipped onto the die. The patient waits while the wax pattern is developed using the molten wax as previously described. Since the facial surface will be shaped to ideal contours, the patient will not be needed again until the crown is completed and the repair clasp added. At this time, the crown is cemented and the partial seated. Occasionally, despite one's best efforts, some adjustment of either the casting or the clasp is required. Again, Mylar tape is the method of choice for identifying points of premature contact. Since the clasp will be made of wire, and as often as possible in the I-bar form, the adjustment of the clasp is not difficult.

Relines and Rebases

Periodic relining of the distal extension areas of the removable partial denture is an essential component of the maintenance phase of therapy. Relines of recent extraction areas are also required. The clinician is faced with deciding between a laboratory reline and one done at the chair. Unlike complete dentures, where a laboratory reline is preferable in all but very temporary situations, the partial denture reline is best done in the mouth. The reason for this difference lies in the fact that the partial denture casting has a different relationship to the abutment teeth when it is being relined in a flask than when it was originally processed.

When the partial denture is processed in the denture flask, it remains on the master cast so that the tooth-frame relation cannot change, even if the technician should not get the flask completely closed when packing the resin. The result of any error here would be a prematurity in the occlusion, which is easy to correct. In a laboratory reline, however, the partial denture does not stay on the cast but ends up in the other half of the flask. Now, when the technician does not get the flask completely closed, the tooth-frame relationship is destroyed and the completed reline will not seat completely onto the abutment teeth.

To avoid any chance of this disaster occurring, a resin that cures either completely or partially in the mouth is used. This allows the clinician to fully seat and maintain the casting on the abutment teeth while the resin polymerizes. The partially light-cured resin, Astron (Anstron Dental, Wheeling, IL) or a similar material, is an excellent choice for the RPD reline, as it is quite color-stable over time; also, because it only partially cures in the mouth, the clinician need not fear locking in place around abutment teeth.

Regardless of which reline approach is chosen, the preparation of the partial denture base for the reline impression is nearly identical. For the reline material (either resin or impression material) to flow freely when the partial is seated on the teeth, the clinician must be certain that adequate space exists between the base and the supporting ridge. Just because the partial denture rocks or the patient complains of movement, it cannot be assumed that a uniform space exists under the base.

To register the tissue-base relation, a thin layer of specially prepared alginate is placed in the base and the denture is seated completely. This alginate is a mixture of one scoop of regular-set alginate with two units of hot water. The resultant mix will be the consistency of soup, so it will not displace tissue but will set quickly because of the hot water. When the partial denture is removed from the mouth, the tissue-base relation is easily seen and any areas of contact are marked before the alginate is removed. The alginate can be torn to evaluate its thickness. Often there will be 1 to 2 mm of space over the ridge, especially in the mandible, but no space will exist in the lingual flange area. The clinician will need to relieve the contact areas so that 1 mm of space, at the very least, is present overall. In some instances, this will mean that the underside of the raised meshwork is completely exposed. This

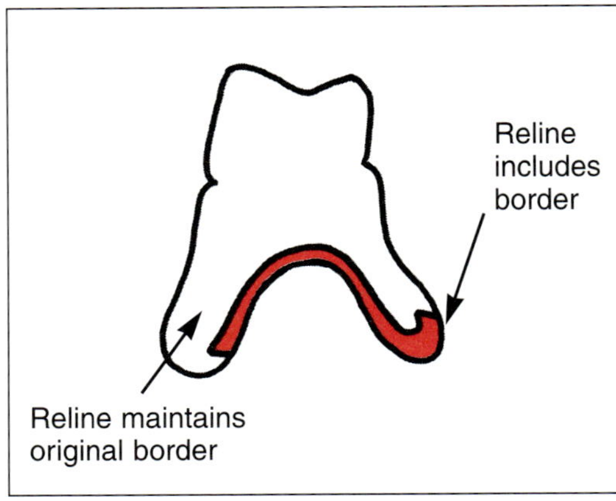

Fig 8-9 Creation of uniform relief after alginate evaluation, with finishing lines.

space is critical for the free flow of the impression material or resin.

A decision must also be made as to the adequacy of the border extensions. The light-cured resin cannot be expected to create a proper border roll if the existing border is underextended more than 3 mm. If the existing borders are greatly underextended, a rebase of the partial denture casting should be considered, which would entail a pick-up impression as described earlier. If the existing borders are properly extended, a finishing line should be cut into the resin border to provide for a butt joint of the new resin with the old. This will reduce the possibility that repair resin will peel away later, which is often the case when a very thin flash of resin exists at the border. The goal of the partial denture reline should be to add a uniform layer of new resin overall (Fig 8-9). The same finishing line should be created for an impression to be used in a laboratory reline if that option is chosen. It will give a positive line for cutting away any excess impression material before pouring the repair cast.

The light-cured reline material will set to a firm but resilient mass in the mouth without the generation of heat but, as with all resin materials, with a strange taste. When inserting the partial into the mouth with the reline resin in place, a small amount of the resin should be placed in the clinician's mouth so that the initial set of the material can be evaluated. When the mass attains the consistency of bubble gum, it is safe to remove the partial denture because the addition is beyond the stage of possible distortion. After trimming any gross excess with scissors (never with a knife), an oxygen barrier is painted on the reline surface and the final cure is made with a light unit. A simple light source such as that used to make trays is perfectly acceptable to complete the cure.

To complete the reline procedure, the clinician must be prepared to adjust the occlusion, especially if the opposing arch is a complete denture. Since the loss of ridge support occurs over an extended period of time, migration of the opposing dentition or prostheses is to be expected. This would require a clinical remount procedure if a complete denture is involved, since intraoral adjustments on unstable bases will never give the quality of occlusal contacts that can be developed on the articulator.

While the base support must be evaluated as part of the annual recall examination, the actual need for a reline on a mature ridge should not occur more often than once every 4 to 6 years. When a solid tissue-base relationship exists, concern over the stress relief built into the design of the partial becomes purely academic; rotation of the partial during function can be expected to be within the tolerance of the periodontal membrane, thus eliminating destructive torquing of the abutment teeth.

As part of the recall evaluation, the wear of the occlusal surfaces of the denture teeth must be evaluated and the addition of metal considered. As discussed earlier, it may be appropriate to evaluate the wear potential of the resin teeth over a period of time and only convert to metal when a total lack of contact is found. Conversion to metal is best done immediately after the reline of the denture base(s).

Given what we now know about the need for continual maintenance of even our best efforts, the repairs, additions, and relines of all types of removable partial dentures become a critical component of the state-of-the-art partial denture. Even though we have made every effort to design and construct the strongest possible partials, we know that we will be required to perform these services, with the help of our technicians, on a routine basis, along with equal efforts in combating caries and periodontal disease.

9

Special Prostheses

There are three special modifications of the partial denture we are trying to create that are different enough to merit a special chapter. The strut rest has proven to be a valuable tool in the support of multiple abutments with compromised bony support. The hinged partial denture offers a means of managing failing or severely compromised dentitions almost to the last tooth, and the rotational path of insertion partial permits the esthetic replacement of missing anterior teeth in most Class IV situations.

Splinting with the RPD

The use of the removable partial denture to support multiple teeth with mobility has long been questioned. Certainly, fixed prostheses offer a more dependable means of joining loose teeth into a single unit. There will be situations, however, when the removable partial will be called upon to offer maximum support to the remaining teeth, either for financial reasons or because of the number of missing teeth in the arch. The best treatment for these situations is obviously some combination of fixed and removable prostheses where ideal contours—guiding planes and rest preparations—can be created on all remaining teeth. Careful, well-planned mouth preparation of multiple teeth, coupled with ideal casting control, can offer excellent support to weakened dentitions and has been shown to actually reduce mobility over time.

To achieve these results, special mouth preparation is required. Perhaps the most common modification of conventional preparation is the use of the "strut" or continuous occlusal rest preparation. Instead of a series of multiple regular occlusal rests, this continuous rest runs from tooth to tooth as a channel in the center of the occlusal surface of the remaining teeth and is joined to a proximal guide plate at either end of the block of contacting teeth. The channel needs to have a width of 3 mm and a depth of 1.2 mm for adequate strength

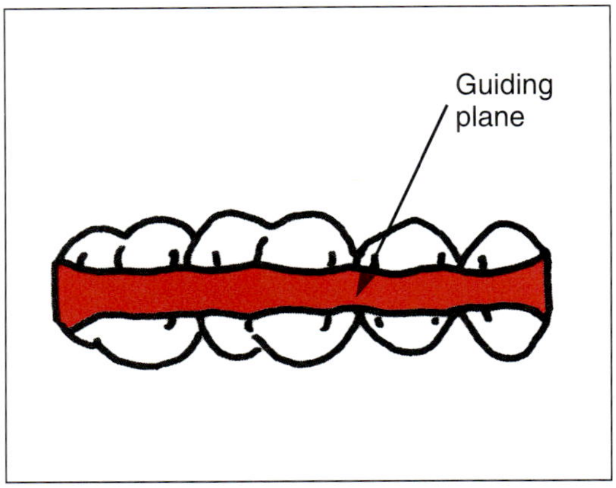

Fig 9-1 Design of continuous or "strut" rest with terminal guiding planes.

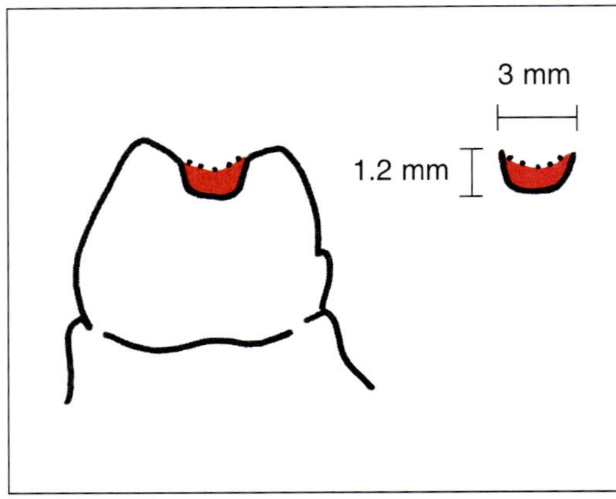

Fig 9-2 Cross section of continuous rest.

(Fig 9-1). The buccal and lingual sides of the preparation must be slightly tapered, with rounded internal angles to facilitate a complete seating of the partial. These surfaces must draw with the prepared guiding plane surfaces and therefore must be reevaluated during the surveying of the check cast before final impressions (Fig 9-2). When an extension of this rest is placed on the last tooth in the arch, normally a second molar, this amount of metal will create a rigid rest despite the cantilever from a more anterior tooth.

Since the rest will be in occlusion with the opposing arch along its total length, some modification of the waxing technique is required to minimize the amount of occlusal adjustment on this very hard alloy. The laboratory can mount the refractory cast and wax directly to the opposing occlusion, or the rest can be waxed on a mounted master cast and transferred to the refractory during the final waxing of the partial. The advantage of the latter technique is that it allows the clinician to create the desired occlusion on the master cast rather than try to describe it to the technician. When waxing the occlusal strut to be transferred, a hard wax should be used to reduce distortion during removal from the lubricated cast and its placement on the refractory. After finishing, the surface of this special rest should be sandblasted so that any eccentric interferences to a smooth disclusion can be easily identified during the first few days of wear. After the adjustment period, the final polish can be easily restored using rubber points and a rag wheel with appropriate polishing compounds.

When this special rest is properly constructed, it will stabilize loose teeth both in centric occlusion and in eccentric movements. This is because the teeth cannot move independently from the partial when it is fully seated with ideal tooth-frame contact. While this rest may not be "esthetic," it normally appears as a series of occlusal amalgams to the eye of the patient. Anterior teeth involved with this type of splinting will require positive rests, either cingulum or incisal, to maintain the tooth-frame relationship during occlusal loading. Simply plating the lingual surfaces will not serve to "splint" mobile teeth.

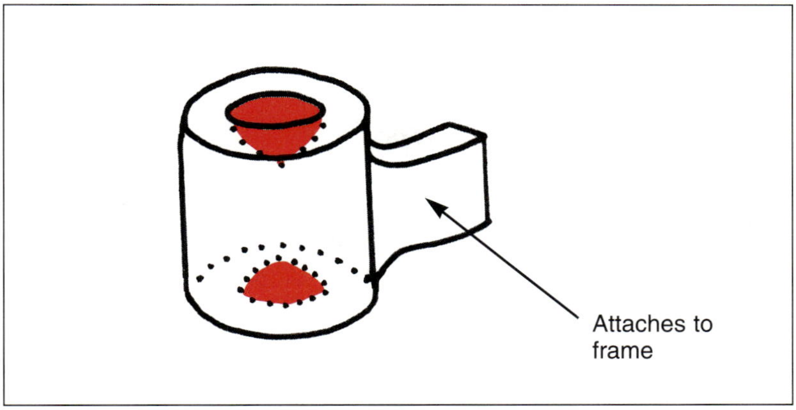

Fig 9-3 Designof hinge.

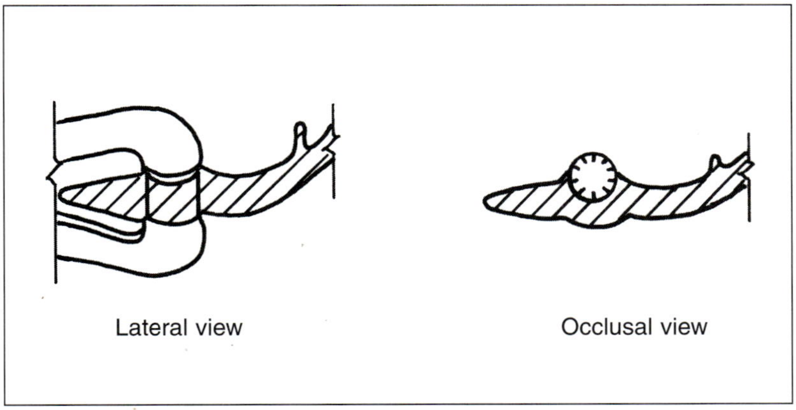

Fig 9-4 Design of latch.

Hinged Major Connectors

The hinged major connector, commonly referred to as a "Swinglock" (actually a patented name and technique), is another special prosthesis that offers excellent splinting capabilities as well as a means of retention when normal tooth contours are not available for any reason. A barrel-shaped hinge with retaining dimples is attached to the major connector with a minor connector that will, in most instances, exit from an edentulous area (Fig 9-3). On the opposite side of the arch, a retaining latch of some sort extends in a similar fashion via a minor connector (Fig 9-4). Connecting these two terminals is a bar with projections to the gingival enamel of the enclosed teeth that swings from the hinge and snaps into the latch. When the prosthesis is in the closed and latched position, all the enclosed teeth are locked together (Fig 9-5). The bar portion can take many forms, one of the popular options being a plate that runs from the vestibule to just incisal to the dentoenamel junction. The outer surface of the plate has a gingival finishing line and microbead retention for a thin resin veneer (Fig 9-6). When the plate is opaqued with the proper shade and suitably colored with resin stains, this gingival apron blends in as natural gingiva.

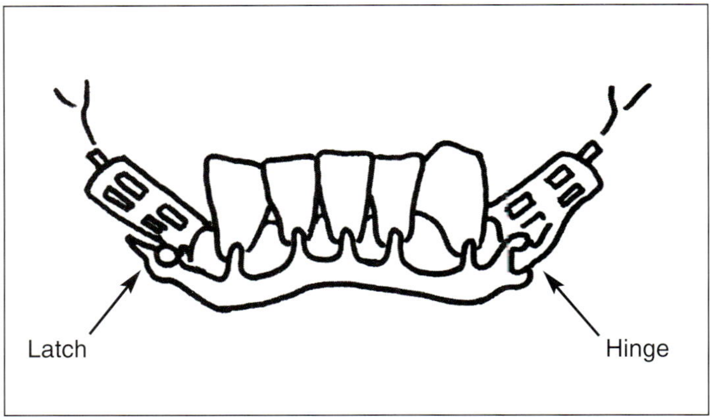

Fig 9-5 Frontal view of hinged major connector.

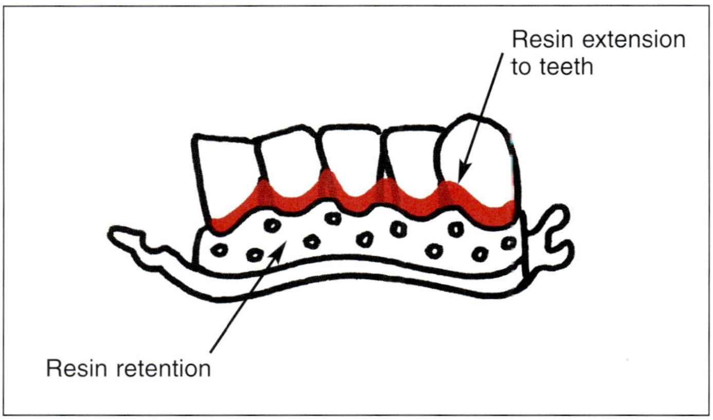

Fig 9-6 Veneered labial plate.

The laboratory has two options for constructing the hinge/latch combination. The most common technique uses the patented components, hinge and latch, which are added to the wax-up of the partial and retained in the casting by means of retentive contours in the metal. A more sophisticated and potentially more precise approach involves two castings. The first casting contains the basic structures of the partial denture and the hinge and latch. After this section has been cast and finished, it is returned to the master cast and reduplicated; the casting remains in the duplicating agar and the refractory material is poured against it. On this second refractory, the bar component is waxed to the hinge and latch. It is sprued and "cast to" the first casting (Fig 9-7). A precise hinge and latch results, since the freedom of movement is created by the thickness of the oxide layer that forms on the first casting when it is placed in the furnace to burn out the second (bar segment) refractory. Using this technique, it is possible to make smaller and more precise joints than one can achieve with commercial components.

The Swinglock concept was originally presented as a technique requiring no mouth preparation of any kind. Subsequent clinical studies have demonstrated that rest preparations are needed to assure that the

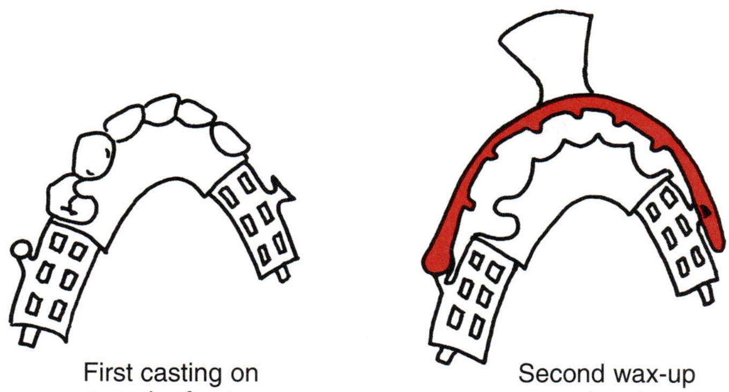

Fig 9-7 Double casting for hinged connector.

entire assembly does not slip gingivally on the teeth. Since the hinged gate effectively holds all the teeth it touches in contact with the main casting, mesial migration of these teeth will not occur. A single, positive rest form of any type on each side of the casting will keep it from settling. The hinged prosthesis has the same requirements for the management of any distal extension base (especially on the mandible). Since these castings are far more complex than the standard partial denture framework, the clinician can expect to be charged a fee 75% to 100% higher than for a routine partial denture casting.

The hinged appliance has two major indications. The most common use is in compromised mandibular situations where only a few anterior teeth remain. When one or both of the mandibular canines is missing, it is often next to impossible to obtain adequate retention by clasping a lateral incisor. In these situations, the remaining teeth are often compromised periodontally, which makes splinting them into one multirooted abutment advisable. It is critical, however, to provide a positive rest seat on the terminal abutment on either side to eliminate the possibility of settling. The other indication, found far less often, is for maxillary situations where the remaining teeth are all on the same side of the arch, often in a more or less straight line. This situation is often found in maxillofacial patients who have lost half of the maxilla as the result of a maxillary tumor. The splinting effect of joining all the remaining teeth is often the only means of supporting and maintaining the prosthesis.

Special problems exist for the hinged appliance that are not found in the routine partial denture situation. There must be enough of a buccal vestibule remaining for the labial bar. When this space is minimal, the bar may have to be changed to a veneered plate in order to have sufficient strength. The labial bar is sometimes objectionable to the patient because of the bulk in the lip. The only alternatives to the use of the hinged appliance for these compromised situations are splinted, full-coverage restorations of all remaining teeth with at-

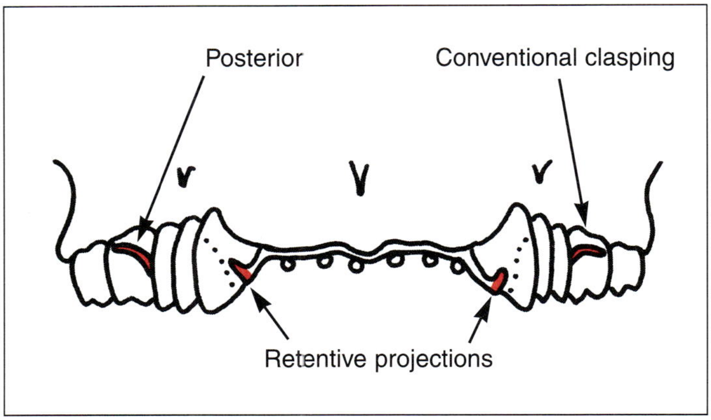

Fig 9-8 Rotational path partial casting fully seated.

tachments, the use of implants, or some combination of the two. Some elderly patients who are compromised by arthritic changes in their hands will have trouble opening and closing the lock mechanism and will require both training and patience to be able to utilize this design. In some extreme situations it may be necessary to remove the gate and replace it with some form of light wire clasping, even though this may be unesthetic and provide only limited retention.

Rotational Partial Dentures

The rotational path of insertion partial denture is a special prosthesis normally used in maxillary Class IV situations where anterior visible clasping is objectionable. This special design utilizes rigid projections into mesial proximal undercuts on the prime abutments (those adjacent to the anterior edentulous space) to retain the anterior part of the partial (Fig 9-8). Since these projections are not clasps, in that they do not flex, they must be placed into the undercuts by inserting the partial first in the anterior and then rotating the posterior of the casting to place; the rigid projections act as the rotational point(s), hence the name "rotational partial denture" (Fig 9-9). Because the posterior part of the casting must be rotated to place, any projections that might interfere with the rotation must be eliminated from the design. This usually implies that there be no modification spaces in the posterior segments and that the major connector be open from the rest in the anterior to the posterior minor connector for the posterior clasp (Fig 9-10). If the modification spaces were present, the additional potential guiding plane surfaces, properly utilized, would make the rotational design unnecessary because anterior clasping would not be required.

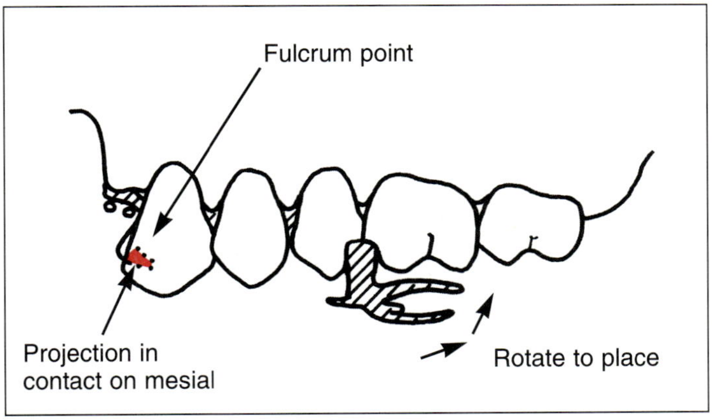

Fig 9-9 Anterior component seated, before rotation.

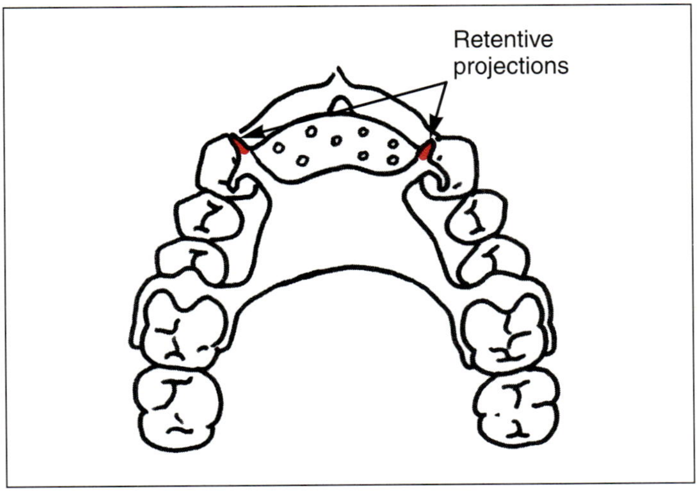

Fig 9-10 Class IV rotational partial, occlusal view.

The prime abutment teeth must have well-defined, positive rest preparations. Any movement of these teeth over time will result in the possible loss of the partial's retention as well as in its inability to completely seat onto the abutment teeth. This design provides anterior retention, since when the partial is fully seated, the anterior segment cannot rotate down and out of the mouth due to the rigid projections in the anterior undercuts. The posterior part of the casting is held in place by embrasure clasps on either the first or second molar, bilaterally. The positive rests on the prime abutments provide a solid stop against movement toward the tissue. The result is a retentive partial that replaces anterior teeth without the show of clasps in the front of the mouth.

The projection into the proximal undercut can take the form of a clasp-like arm if the tooth involved is an anterior, or a part of the minor connector if the prime abutment is a premolar (Fig 9-11). Special care must be taken in the laboratory to ensure that this projection is in no way altered, either in the blockout (of which there should be none under the projection) or in the electrolytic

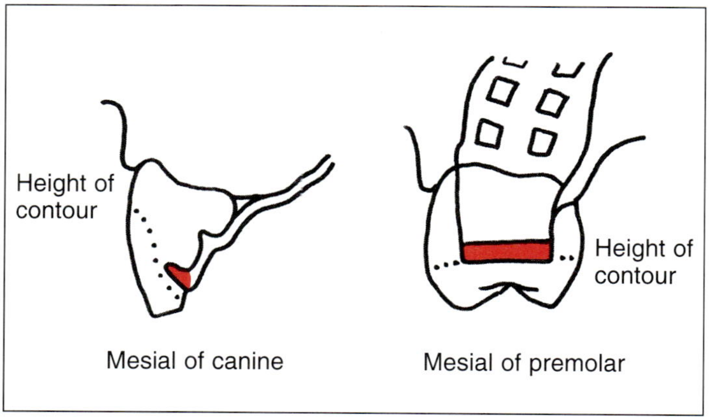

Fig 9-11 Rotational elements, no blockout.

stripping and finishing of the metal. This projection must contact the tooth for the retention of the anterior segment to be acceptable; therefore, the casting must be fitted first to the mouth and then placed on the cast without regard to possibly scraping the cast. The clinician can expect to find interferences to the rotation of the casting. These must be identified and adjusted intraorally using some form of disclosing material. Care must be taken when adjusting the rigid projections; as opposed to a clasp, they will be too short and rigid to bring into tooth contact.

Since the anterior segment must be rotated into place, the anterior flange can only extend to the height of contour of the edentulous ridge and must be tapered to a very thin margin to avoid creating a ledge that will accumulate food (Fig 9-12). In cases of anterior ridge destruction there may be no anterior undercut. In this situation, the flange is fully extended to provide lip support and the resin retention of choice is a raised retentive mesh, since any large soft tissue defect can be expected to eventually need a reline. In mature ridges without loss of contour, the metal base with suitable retentive devices for the denture teeth is preferred. Depending on where the metal of the casting ends on the facial gingiva, the casting may require opaquing and tinting of the denture base. Since the resin in the labial flange will most always be on the thin side, some experimentation with the tinting will be required. There will not be the normal depth of denture base resin to back up the tints and, as a result, the colors will not appear as one would expect from the tinting of a standard denture base.

It is also possible to reverse the rotation direction by placing the rotation points in the posterior of the mouth. This design has been advocated in the literature for Class III mandibular partial dentures where the posterior abutments have migrated mesially, leaving large proximal undercuts. Rigid, cast metal is extended into these mesial undercut areas and the partial is rotated to place on that axis. No guiding plane is possible on the distal aspect of the anterior abutments, so retentive clasping is required on these

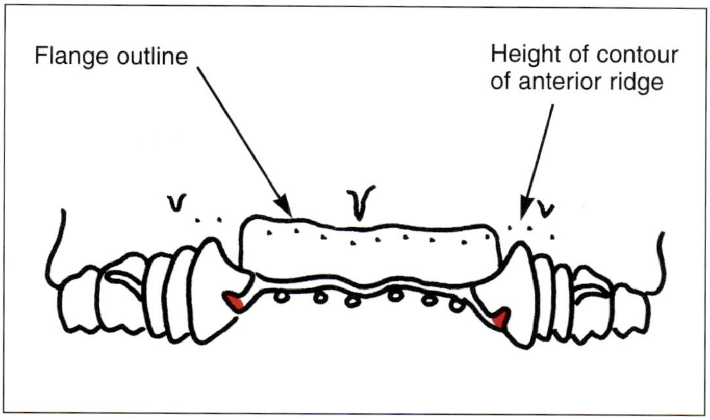

Fig 9-12 Flange extension for Class IV rotational partial.

teeth. There is no disadvantage, either functional or esthetic, to posterior clasping, so I see no advantage to this design and cannot recommend it.

The patient will often require some extra time and instruction in the placement and removal of the rotational path partial. While some loss of retention over time can be expected, the amount of actual wear from the friction of rotation is really minimal so that the partial should be serviceable for a normal period of wear.

10

Precision Attachments

The precision attachment denture has long been considered the highest form of partial denture therapy. It combines fixed and removable prosthodontics in such a way as to create the most esthetic partial possible. It also has the reputation of lasting far longer than the conventional partial. What possible biological reason could exist to support this reputation? It has long been my belief that the reason this prosthesis is, in general, so successful is that the clinician and the laboratory simply must take greater pains in every aspect of construction just to get the precision attachment partial into the mouth. Since the cost of this particular therapy is apt to be far greater than for a conventional partial denture, there is a greater likelihood of long-term follow-up care and high-quality maintenance. If the more conventional partial denture, one that is clasp-retained, is constructed as described in this text, there is no inherent reason that the attachment-retained partial should be superior.

The precision attachment partial should differ only in the means of its retention when compared to the clasp-retained partial denture. The only reason for utilizing this mechanical device is to replace the visible clasp arm. All other functions of the partial can be performed by conventional means if they are understood and the partial is constructed to the highest standards.

Until just the last few years, the use of a precision attachment required the construction of one or more crowns as part of the treatment. With the advent of resin-bonded metal components, a whole new era has opened for the attachment-retained partial. The demand for what might be called "fashion magazine" esthetics, so apparent in our modern society, has made many of our patients unwilling to accept visible anterior clasping, and so we see an increasing need to offer this type of prosthesis. The combination of these two seemingly unrelated statements will create a demand for a more sophisticated partial denture, one in which good tooth structure will not have to be sacrificed to allow maximum esthetics.

Since the construction of the precision attachment partial denture is technically demanding, the need for the clinician to fully understand the implications for the dental laboratory is critical to success. It is to that end that the subject is presented in some detail in this chapter. The sheer number of attachments on the market makes a truly comprehensive evaluation next to impossible. A solid understanding of the use of six basic categories of attachments will provide the clinician with tools to evaluate other attachment systems as they come on the market and to choose those that offer the greatest potential for long-term success.

Common Clinical Procedures

A number of clinical procedures common to the use of any attachment system must be mastered before a real level of confidence can be achieved.

Diagnostic Procedures

Space will almost always be a major consideration and a problem for precision attachment selection and use; therefore, a diagnostic wax-up and set-up is essential for every case. Regardless of what is found in the opposing arch, this diagnostic positioning of teeth on bases that will allow verification in the mouth must be done so that tooth position can be evaluated, both by the clinician and the patient. The final position of all teeth and the denture base must be known to ensure that the space requirements of the attachment system under consideration can be met. When insufficient space is available, either the system selected or the oral environment must change, through surgeries, orthodontics, or tooth modification. The clinician will need an up-to-date, comprehensive catalog of attachment systems that indicates all dimensions of each unit. In choosing an attachment system, the laboratory must be a willing collaborator; it must have experience with the chosen system or be willing to experiment along with the clinician. Attachments International, the Preat Corporation, APM-Sterngold, and Cendres & Metaux all have current catalogs, most of which contain technical guidance as well as precise descriptions of a wide variety of attachment systems. These catalogs should be available, in a current edition, from the dental laboratory.

The Pick-up Impression

The clinician must develop a technique for making a final impression for the removable partial denture framework that includes picking up the completed fixed components from the mouth in such a way that the position of the units remains accurately related to the remainder of the mouth. Having the actual crowns on the master cast allows precise positioning of the attachment components, a task that may not be possible when working on a stone replica of the crown, due to the probable fracturing of thin projections of stone. It also allows the master cast to be used as a milling cast to provide a stable platform for milling metal surfaces of the fixed components. This procedure will require a custom impression tray and an impression made with a relatively rigid material, usually a silicone or a polyether. The fixed units will have to be completely retentive on the tooth because of the inherent fit of the casting, or, if there is a potential for movement during the master impression, they will have to be temporarily cemented to keep them from moving. The cementing medium for this procedure must be one that will allow the unit to be removed from the mouth with the final impression, since replacing a unit in an elastic material runs the risk of creating an inaccurate relationship. A small bead of Fit-Checker, placed just internal to the margin, will usually maintain the casting-tooth relationship. An equally small bead of Temp-Bond (Kerr, Romulus, MI) with Vaseline also can be used. When the impression is removed from the mouth and is found to be acceptable, resin dies that have been made previously are placed into each fixed unit, and the impression is boxed and poured.

These dies are made with an autopolymerizing resin, such as Duralay (Reliance Dental, Worth, IL), with a retentive wire projection to lock them into the dental stone of the master cast (Fig 10-1). The completed crown is lubricated and the resin is added up to the margin. A wire that has been serrated is inserted into the resin mass, and the resin is allowed to set. The portion of the wire that protrudes from the crown is bent into some retentive form to retain it in the stone. The crown must seat completely on the resin die with the margin protected and be easily removed from the cast as needed. This is particularly true if the crown has a porcelain butt margin. The master cast must always be poured in improved die stone to gain maximum resistance to fracture and abrasion.

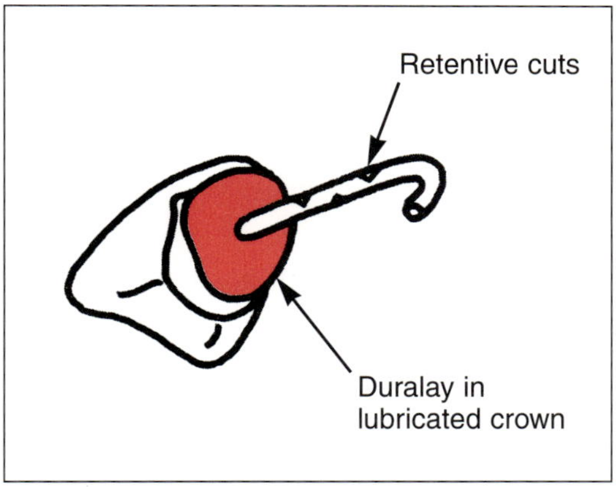

Fig 10-1 Pick-up die with wire retention.

A very real potential exists for fracturing any porcelain butt margins that may be present when the impression is removed from the master cast. For this reason, the impression tray must always be custom-made of regular laboratory tray material. These resins, unlike those that are light activated, can be heated with an alcohol torch and softened enough to peel the tray off the cast without fear of damaging the fixed components. Stock metal trays, perfectly adequate for most framework impressions, will obviously not offer this option and should not be used. Once the tray is removed, the impression material can be easily separated from the cast.

Pick-up of Attachment Components

The clinician, with the aid of the chairside assistant, must develop a technique for joining attachment components to the framework directly in the mouth as well as on the cast. With the advent of light-activated resins, such as Palavit GLC from Kulzer, the clinician can maintain the appropriate position of the various components while the assistant places the resin and activates it with the light. If any load is to be placed on the attachment during removal from the mouth, a used dental bur can be added to the composite mass to strengthen it. Each attachment system will require slightly different pick-up techniques, requiring some level of experience to routinely join the attachment to the casting without introducing error. In many instances, it may be appropriate to join the attachment to the framework out on the bench. Generally speaking, it is easier to make a quality resin bond on the bench and then take it back to the mouth to verify the accuracy of the relationship. These steps of verification are essential to success with precision attachments. Some attachments, such as clips for bar-clip attachments, will be picked up using a laboratory autocuring resin having the same coloration as the denture base.

Other attachment systems will require that some portion of the unit, either the matrix or patrix, be joined to the removable partial denture casting in the mouth. The same approach as was used for certain types of repair impressions will be needed. In other words, the clinician must relate the components while an auxiliary places the resin and cures the mass. As with the repair, either an autopolymerizing resin like Duralay or a light-cured resin like Palavit can be used. The light-cured resin is more expensive but quicker to use. Attachment systems can be soldered to the framework or joined in resin alone, the choice depending primarily on the amount of available space and the possible need for retrievability. When space is at a premium, the soldering option is definitely the technique of choice.

In addition to these specific techniques, altered cast impressions and precise jaw relation recording systems must be available for the construction of the precision attachment partial denture. The altered cast impression will be made after the attachment system has been joined to the framework, since the object of the altered cast is to record the support of the soft tissue in relation to the abutment teeth through the fit of the casting. Adding the attachments after the altered cast impression could alter this tissue-tooth relationship if any movement of components occurs.

Crown Preparation for Intracoronal Attachments

When intracoronal attachments are to be used, the preparation design for the abutment tooth will have to be modified from that of a standard full-veneer crown preparation. To create a crown that has normal emergence profiles and dimensions, some form of box preparation that will relate to the dimensions of the chosen attachment must be made. A review of pulpal anatomy is essential to preclude overpreparation of the abutment tooth. This may require the preparation on the bench of extracted teeth with dimensions similar to those of the actual abutment tooth. The presence of secondary dentin and the determination of its depth become critical issues. When considering the preparation depth, the minimum thickness of the alloy, usually around 0.5 mm, must be added to the dimensions of the attachment matrix. If this reduction places the tooth at risk for overpreparation, the choice of attachment sys-

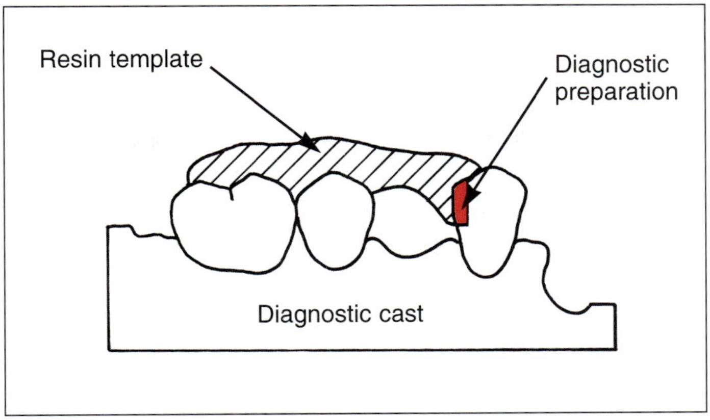

Fig 10-2 Preparation guide for intracoronal attachment.

tem must be reevaluated. The use of an extracoronal attachment instead of an intracoronal is an obvious solution to the problem.

The stone tooth representing the abutment on the diagnostic cast must be prepared to accept the matrix plus the minimum space necessary for the gold of the crown. The matrix can be tried in place on the prepared tooth using the holding device that fits into the dental surveyor and, once adequate space has been created, a template can be quickly constructed that will transfer the preparation form to the mouth. The prepared stone tooth and the occlusal surfaces of adjacent teeth are painted with an alginate-based separating agent, and an autopolymerizing resin is placed into the cavity and onto the occlusal surfaces of the adjacent teeth (Fig 10-2). When set, the template can be trimmed of excess resin and taken to the mouth to verify the dimensions of the matrix cavity by placing it onto the adjacent teeth and modifying the preparation until it accepts the form. The use of this simple preparation guide reduces the risk of overpreparation of the tooth and guarantees that there has been enough reduction to allow the matrix to be placed within the normal contours of the abutment tooth.

Converting an Existing Cast RPD to a Provisional Resin RPD

One of the most difficult tasks the clinician will face in the construction of a precision attachment partial denture is maintaining the patient's existing partial throughout what may be a long treatment time. When orthodontics and perhaps even orthognathic surgery are involved in addition to implants, treatment time can extend to years. Trying to make quality provisional fixed restorations that will support an existing removable partial denture for that length of time may well be impossible. It is in the best interests of the clinician as well as the patient to convert an existing metal-frame partial denture to a quality resin appliance made in conjunction with any re-

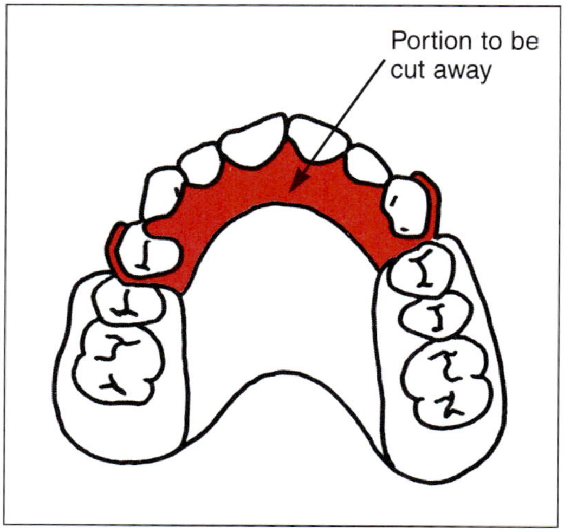

Fig 10-3 Preparation of an old RPD for conversion to a provisional removable appliance.

quired fixed provisional restorations. While there are many ways of creating these provisionals, it is important to bear in mind the cost to the patient. The following technique creates a quality long-term provisional at minimum cost to the patient.

The first step is to prepare the existing partial denture for a special type of pick-up impression. Any component of the partial that contacts the remaining teeth is cut away with a large cut-off disc, leaving at least 2 to 3 mm of space between the partial and the teeth (Fig 10-3). This will allow the impression material full access to the teeth. A high-viscosity polyether or silicone impression material is mixed and placed in the partial. The partial is carried to place and maintained in a position of maximum occlusion with the opposing arch, without regard to the abutment teeth, until set. Before removing the partial denture, a second impression, alginate this time, in a stock dentate tray (preferably sectional), is made over the partial and the remainder of the denture-bearing area. Special care is taken to ensure that alginate is wiped onto all remaining teeth and into the space created between the partial and the teeth when the framework was sectioned.

The two impressions are removed together and poured in yellow stone. When the alginate portion of the impression is removed from the cast, the elastomeric impression inside the old partial is left in place until the cast has been mounted in the articulator with the opposing cast. Once the mounting is complete, the partial denture is carefully removed from the cast, leaving the impression material in the partial. At this time, any diagnostic waxing for the fixed provisional component is done according to standard techniques. Rest preparations and guiding planes are prepared, and undercuts ideal for infrabulge I-bar clasps are created. Once the waxing is complete, that cast is duplicated and the partial denture replaced on the duplicate cast.

Flanges are cut away from the partial to create space for the retentive wire bar clasps. These clasps are adapted using Ni-Cr-Co wires and waxed into place on the cast. Additional wax is added to complete the desired form of the provisional partial denture. Since the resin provisional will need to be thicker than the old framework, at least one thickness of baseplate wax must be added to all areas of bare framework. The outline of the provisional will necessarily cover a greater portion of the mouth than did the old metal-based partial (Fig 10-4). For the mandibular provisional, special care must be taken to wax the lingual plate area of the major connector to provide for adequate strength in the resin. Because the pick-up impression was made in maximum occlusal contact, there is no need to articulate this processing cast.

The completed waxed partial is placed in the first half of the processing flask in a normal manner. The second half of the flasking is the key to making this technique possible. The exposed denture with its added wax contours is covered with an elastomeric mold release material (Dent-kote from Dentsply or a material of similar weight). Immediately after placing this material, usually with the finger to assure that no voids are created, the second half of the flasking is completed using the normal mix of dental stone. This immediate pouring of the stone onto the as-yet not set silicone is essential to keep them from separating during the boilout and opening of the flask.

When the flasking stone is set, the flask is boiled out in the normal manner. When the flask is opened, the old partial is easily removed from the mold. After completing the boil-out, the cast is painted with separator. A small amount of autopolymerizing resin is added to the tang of the bar clasps to stabilize them during packing. The reason for selecting the infrabulge clasps for this provisional denture should now be apparent. Had a normal circumferential clasp been used, it would have had to cross the occlusal surface of the partial, which might have made removing the old partial from the flask a difficult task.

If the denture teeth from the old partial are porcelain, they can be removed from the denture bases by warming the base resin with a Hanau torch and prying them from the softened mass of resin. They are cleaned and placed back in their cavities in the silicone mold release material. Resin denture teeth will normally be found, since porcelain teeth are seldom used for partial dentures. The technician has the option of cutting the resin teeth and their associated denture base material from the old partial

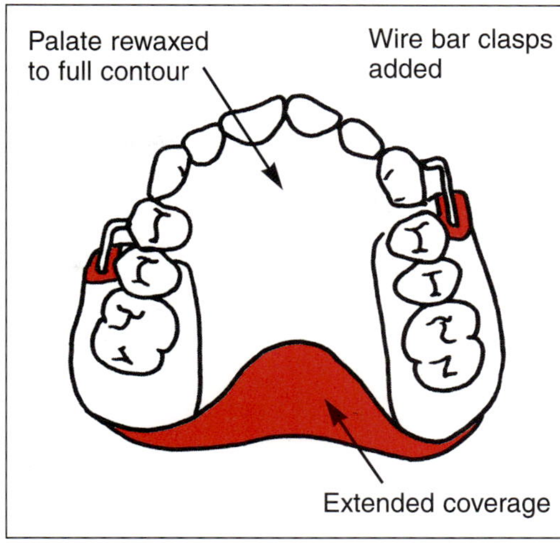

Fig 10-4 Final waxing of converted cast partial denture.

in a block and placing it back in the mold or pouring tooth-colored resin into the tooth negatives in the elastomeric material. The flask would then be placed in a pressure pot for the cure of the new denture teeth. The segment of teeth will have to be taken out of the mold and the excess resin removed before placing it back into the mold for final processing. In either case, the provisional partial is packed in a high-impact, heat-cured resin and processed and finished in the normal manner.

The original master cast, with its waxed provisional restoration, is now used to create an eggshell fixed provisional for relining in the mouth. Additional wax is added to the marginal one third of the teeth to be provisionalized to assure adequate resin at the margin, and a putty mold of the wax-up is made. Tooth-colored resin of the appropriate shade is painted into the putty, usually with both incisal and body resin, and the mold is placed in the pressure pot. Since the fixed provisional restoration will be required to support the removable pro-

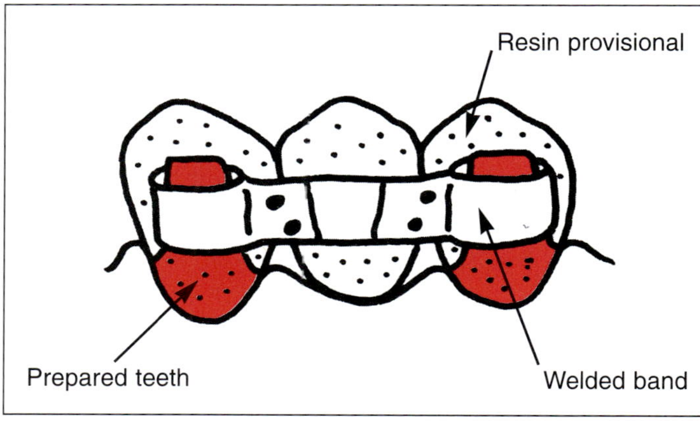

Fig 10-5 Fixed provisional reinforced with welded orthodontic band material.

visional, the stresses placed on the temporary cement seal will be greatly increased, especially if the provisional partial is a Class I and can rotate in function. Any washout of cement and resultant caries will create a disaster that can be at least partially overcome by reinforcing the provisional with orthodontic band material. The band material is loosely adapted to the preparation and spot welded in the interproximal areas as well as in the edentulous pontic areas. When completely adapted, the band is placed in the mouth and the fixed provisional shell is relined in normal fashion, resulting in a metal-reinforced provisional fixed unit that has a greatly increased resistance to flexure and cement seal fracture (Fig 10-5).

Since the fixed provisionals and the removable provisional partial denture were made from the same master cast, they will, with a minimum of adjustment, fit together. In fact, it is in this state that the relining of the fixed provisionals onto the prepared teeth will occur. To reline the fixed provisionals without regard to the removable partial will almost assure that their relationship will change and that unnecessary adjustments to the resin partial will be required to seat the removable provisional restoration. Rather than completely fill the fixed provisional restorations with resin to reline them, only a small amount of resin should be placed in the eggshell, and then the entire provisional assembly, fixed and removable, is seated and directed to place using the occlusion with the opposing dentition as the guide for proper placement. The small addition of resin will imprint the occlusal/incisal portion of the prepared teeth and positively relate the provisional. The removable provisional can now be removed from the fixed units and the relining of the fixed provisionals completed without the interference of the removable partial.

The result of all this will be a combined fixed and removable provisional restoration that can be adjusted and added to as needed while other forms of mouth preparation are made. The only chair time expended will be that needed to make the double pick-up impression, so the cost to the patient and clinician will be low. The only downside of this provisional combination will be the added bulk of the all-resin removable portion when compared to the old metal partial denture. Patients generally tolerate this bulk when they know that it will only be temporary.

Immediate Temporary Resin RPDs

Many of the patients whose ultimate treatment will be some form of a precision attachment partial denture with associated fixed prosthesis enter our practices with failing restorations, some fixed and some removable. They are in immediate need of a provisional restoration to carry them through the initial phases of treatment. Often a failing fixed partial denture will present with the loss of retention of one abutment, leaving it supported by only one abutment. The patient is well aware that the fixed partial is loose. The first step in treating such a patient will be to obtain the best possible initial impression of the affected arch. Any attempt to remove the defective fixed partial denture without a usable initial cast of the arch can lead to a major problem if the defective restoration is completely undermined with decay and it is not possible to maintain it in place for a later impression. The patient is without the fixed partial, and a conventional provisional partial denture, especially if a large number of teeth are involved, is some days away from completion.

An almost instant replacement can be made using a combination of autopolymerizing tooth-colored resin, orthodontic resin, and nonprecious I-bar wire clasps. When the original alginate impression is removed from the cast, teeth that will need replacing are poured immediately in the appropriate tooth-colored resin, and the alginate is placed in the pressure pot. The block of teeth is removed and trimmed, and the stone teeth are removed from the cast. Wire clasps, again preferably in the I-bar form, are adapted and waxed to place with sticky wax. The new resin tooth segment is substituted for the stone teeth, and the ridge is trimmed as for any immediate denture situation. Any obvious undercuts on the lingual surfaces of the teeth to be contacted with the denture base are blocked out with baseplate wax to roughly 90 degrees. After coating the cast with a separating medium, the bulk of the partial is formed in the fine-grained orthodontic resin, either pink or clear, and the entire project is placed in the pressure pot.

The resulting partial denture can be expected to closely approximate the defective restoration in tooth position and arrangement. If the patient requires the extraction of nonrestorable teeth, the teeth are removed and the provisional partial is seated and adjusted as needed. Burlew's Dry Foil is then placed over the sockets. Lynal is added to the partial and it is inserted. The Lynal will act as a soft bandage for the initial healing. The purpose of the Dry Foil is to preclude the Lynal being forced up into the socket. Once the Lynal is into its initial set, the partial can be removed from the mouth and the Dry Foil easily peeled out of the Lynal.

Most immediate provisional partial dentures need only one clasp arm per side. As I-bars, these clasps are much easier to adapt initially and are readily adjusted to the abutment teeth if necessary. Any areas

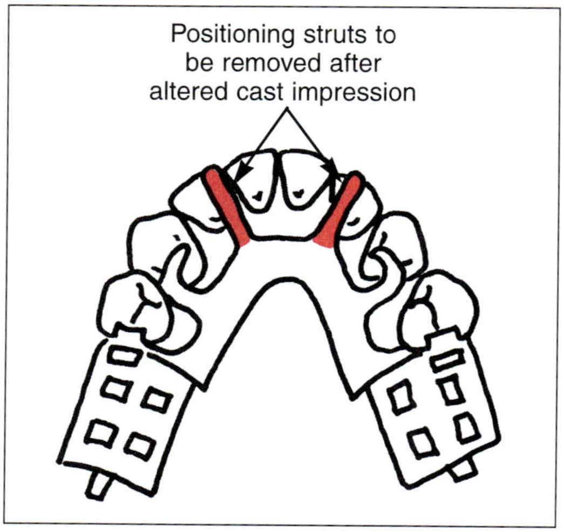

Fig 10-6 Casting modification for precision attachments.

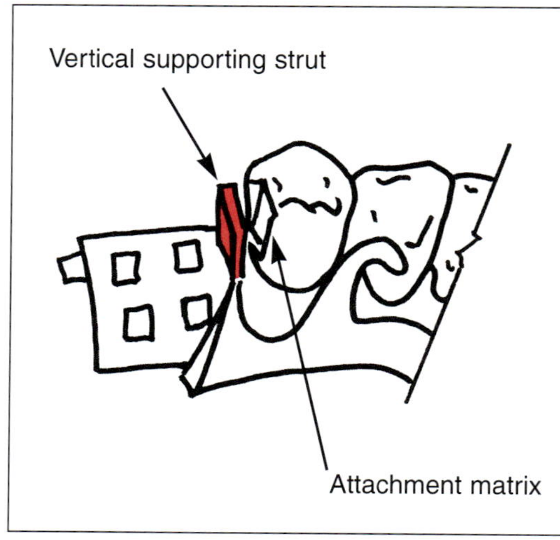

Fig 10-7 Casting modification to support intracoronal attachment.

of this quickly made provisional prosthesis that do not fit satisfactorily can be easily readapted with any autopolymerizing resin intended for oral use.

Modifications of the Framework Design

At times there may not be sufficient contact areas between the framework and the remaining teeth to ensure positive orientation during the pick-up operations described earlier. This will most often be true when attachments that will also bear some of the vertical support of the partial denture are used. In these cases, additional struts are added to the major connector and extend to the occlusal or incisal surface of at least two widely separated teeth (Fig 10-6). The strut is waxed directly on the refractory cast and has the dimensions of a normal minor connector. The struts provide a positive position of the framework in the mouth while attachments are joined to the casting and altered cast impressions are being made. After these two operations are completed and the fit of the attachments is verified, the struts are cut from the major connector and the surface is returned to a normal contour and finish.

Many partial denture frameworks will need a support post added to the resin retention area in order to have something to which the patrix can be either soldered or attached to with resin. The exact shape of this strut will be dependent on the attachment system used, but its design must be reviewed with the laboratory because it is such a critical element (Fig 10-7).

Precision Attachment Systems

Overcoping/Overcrown

The most basic precision attachment system is that of the precision coping. A thin-walled coping cemented in place on the abutment tooth permits an overcoping or overcrown attached to the removable partial denture to fit over it and provide, based on a frictional fit, some degree of retention for the partial denture as well as excellent lateral stability and solid occlusal stop support. These copings are usually milled to the planned path of insertion/removal or with a slight taper, around 2 to 5 degrees, depending on the height of the coping. The height of the coping varies with the crown-root ratio and the integrity of the remaining tooth structure. When very little tooth structure remains, the coping should be used as a stop only, since lateral forces could be unfavorable when precise milling is used. These simple attachments have been used for many years for extensive splinted fixed restorations, commonly referred to as *perioprostheses*, with great success. The entire superstructure can be removed by the patient, providing total access for cleaning. Moreover, should a coping abutment be lost for any reason with time, the tooth can be removed and the overcoping filled with resin to become a pontic. In many cases these large restorations can still be used even with the loss of some of the original abutments. Great success in using this approach for overdentures has also been well-documented.

Obtaining a ferrule effect of at least 1.5 mm on solid tooth structure is critical in the restoration of badly broken down teeth for copings. When endodontically treated teeth are used, this ferrule will dramatically reduce the possibility of root fracture. In many instances, it will be necessary to perform crown-lengthening procedures to gain sufficient tooth structure supragingivally, since the coping margin should be placed at the gingival crest.

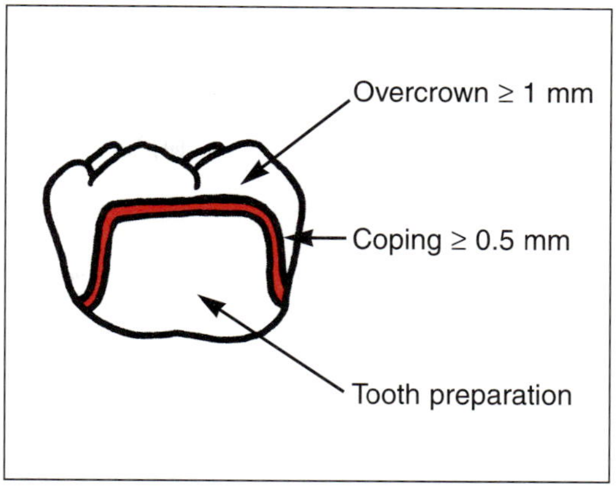

Fig 10-8 Vital tooth coping with overcrown (thickness).

Any posterior tooth or root portion can be considered for a coping restoration. Often, one root of an otherwise periodontally involved molar tooth will have sufficient bone remaining to justify its retention in the mouth. When this root can be maintained, an effective tooth-borne partial denture can be constructed in a situation that would otherwise result in a distal extension base.

Vital abutments, when used with copings, must have sufficient occlusal reduction to allow both the coping and the overcrown to have sufficient thickness to withstand occlusal wear (Fig 10-8). At least

1.5 mm must be available, with the coping needing 0.5 and the crown taking up the remaining space. For this reason, the occlusal surface of the crown should be in metal; porcelain would require at least 2.5 mm of reduction. The need for a facial veneer in the overcrown is a more common requirement. Slightly less than the 2.5-mm space can be used and it will still hold shade and contour. Nonvital abutments are obviously more adaptable to the use of a ceramic overcrown.

The construction of a milled coping starts with a diagnostic wax-up and set-up that will include the opposing arch, be it a complete denture or a partially edentulous restoration. The design of the partial denture is determined and drawn on the diagnostic cast with indications for subtractive mouth preparation. The stone teeth that represent the abutments are prepared for either additive or subtractive mouth preparation to a chosen path of insertion/removal, and the vital abutments that will be used for copings are prepared to the appropriate dimensions and angulations. This diagnostic cast becomes the blueprint for the actual mouth preparation. Endodontically treated abutment teeth usually do not require the same level of diagnostic preparation because there is much more freedom in creating the desired milled contours. After the cast is used as a guide for mouth preparation, it can be used as a prescription for additive mouth preparation by the dental technician. The stone coping teeth are prepared, waxed, and milled on a surveyor using a blade that will attach to the vertical arm of the surveyor. The diagnostic cast will then represent all the desired contours in such a way as to ensure that the technician will be able to reproduce them exactly in the final restorations.

The actual preparation of the coping abutments occurs only after all the subtractive mouth preparation has been completed. In this way, the prepared guiding planes can serve as vertical indicators of the final path of insertion/removal during the preparation of the abutments that will receive copings.

The master impression must involve all the teeth in the arch as well as all edentulous landmarks that will be required for the construction of the final partial denture framework, even though the casting will never be made from this cast. Once the dies have been trimmed and the casts mounted in the articulator, the copings can be rough waxed. The prepared dies are dipped in molten wax to establish a thickness of at least 1 mm and then milled to the desired taper with the dental surveyor or with wax burs in the industrial milling machine, which must be available in the dental laboratory chosen to support the treatment.

When the milling is complete, the waxed copings are marginated to allow for a coping margin of at least 1 mm. The placement of this margin will determine the margin of the overcrown or overcoping. Because of the angulation of an isolated tooth relative to the path of insertion/removal that the partial denture must take, it may not be possible to mill all sides of the coping to that path for the full length of the coping. In such situations, the margin of the overcrown or overcoping will rise or fall according to the milled surface (Fig 10-9). The more surfaces that can be paralleled, however, the more the frictional retention of the partial can be increased.

The coping is then sprued and cast in a type IV gold to reduce long-term wear, finished, and returned to the master cast. The coping should never be thinner than 0.5

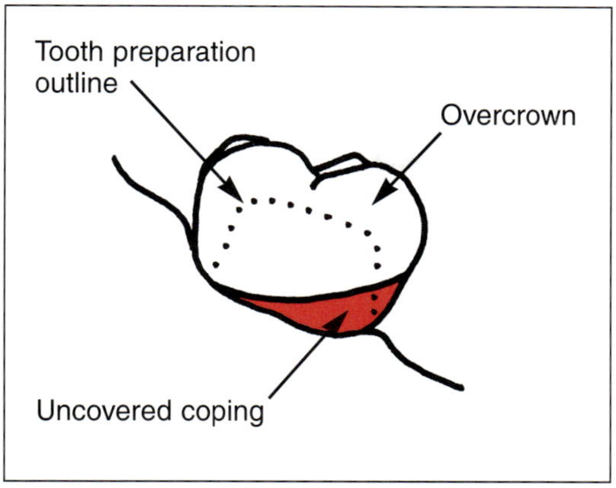

Fig 10-9 Overcrown margin options.

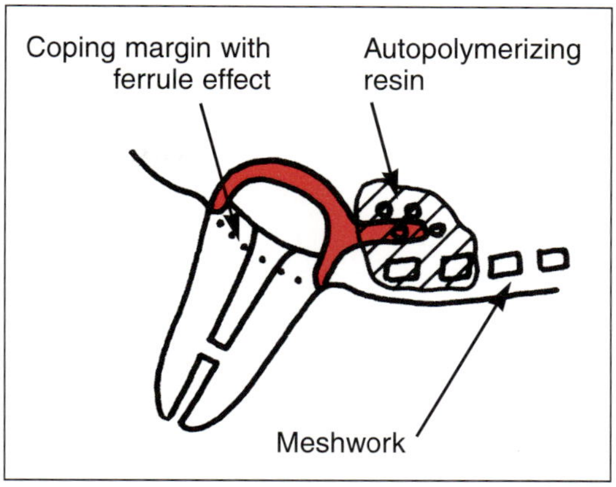

Fig 10-10 Overcoping attached to raised meshwork.

mm in any portion. The copings can now be milled on the milling device to bring them into ideal contour. Great care must be taken in thin areas, obviously, but this should not be a problem in the hands of an experienced technician. The metal is best left in a sandblasted surface; there is no advantage to a high polish, except at the margin with the tooth.

The decision between an overcoping that will have no occlusal anatomy and an overcrown with normal occlusal contours is based on the position of the tooth in the arch and the available interarch space. In general, a second or third molar on the mandibular arch indicates the overcoping as the design of choice if occlusal contacts with the opposing dentition are not essential. The overcrown is then waxed, cast, finished, and veneered if indicated. Both the coping and the overcrown are returned to the mouth so the final impression for the partial denture casting can be made. This impression must pick up the overcrown as it would any additive restoration, since they must all appear on the master cast.

The coping attachment, whether an overcoping or overcrown, will be soldered to the framework in most situations. It is possible to attach retentive loops or beads to the overcoping and retain that unit in the resin base, but the need for this approach is limited to situations where there is a great deal of interocclusal space present and where the extension of the overcrown into occlusion would result in an excessively thick crown (Fig 10-10). These overcrowns can be veneered if they fall into the area where the patient's esthetic demands would be compromised by a full gold crown, but such coping-crown situations are most often found in the posterior part of the mouth where a display of metal is acceptable.

The coping will, in every instance, act as a vertical stop for the partial denture. In most cases it can also provide frictional retention. It is most effective when used in combination with other attachment systems that provide greater resistance to dislodgment or with conventional clasping in other areas of the mouth.

Bar-Clip Attachments

The bar-clip attachment has its origins in turn-of-the-century dentistry, when the Gilmore clip system was made available to the profession. It was commonly used with copings or crowns over vital teeth and later with endodontically treated teeth in which a post coping system attached a solid bar of about 8 gauge to the posts. The attachment mechanism was a plate gold, U-shaped clip, of various lengths, retained in the resin of the prosthesis or soldered to some portion of the internal framework. The Dolder bar system offered an egg-shaped bar that permitted a certain amount of rotation of the prosthesis while still retaining the denture. This system was used extensively in both arches and was equally adaptable to the removable partial denture as the complete denture.

Advances in organic chemistry have resulted in the creation of resilient clips, made of thermoplastic materials, that are very inexpensive and can be rapidly replaced by the clinician. They have the disadvantage of wearing more quickly than the gold plate clips. These plastic clips are offered with a thin metal retainer housing that has retentive contours on the inner surface to retain the clip. They are, in turn, held in the resin of the denture with retentive contours on their outer surface.

Bar-clip systems are widely used with implant-supported overdentures of many different designs and are available from a variety of manufacturers. The bars, in cross section, can be round, pear-shaped, u-shaped, or rectangular. The round and the pear-shaped forms are intended to allow some rotation of the attachment device perpendicular to the long axis of the bar. Among the most popular are the Hader bar, Dolder bar, CM-Rider, and Ackerman clip and bar.

When used as an attachment for a removable partial denture, the bars, either in the form of a castable plastic pattern or as a wrought precious metal bar that is intended to be soldered, are attached to elements of the fixed prosthodontic component. It is again essential that diagnostic wax-ups and set-ups are created to relate the position of the denture teeth to the position of the bar and to assure that adequate space exists—not only for the bar, the clip, and the clip retainer, but for the teeth and associated resin that will usually be placed directly over the bar-clip assembly. When space is limited, the use of a protective metal covering over any thin resin areas is indicated. This will often take the form of a cast-metal occlusal surface for a posterior tooth, since the expected wear of a resin denture tooth in function can result in breakage over the clip assembly.

Once the diagnostic wax-up is complete and the teeth to be replaced on the partial have been tried in the mouth and verified esthetically, a putty matrix of the teeth is made with a positive seat on the cast to allow both the clinician and the technician to find the ideal position for the bar relative to the denture teeth (Fig 10-11). As part of this decision, the vertical position of the bar relative to the soft tissue will have to be selected. If the bar is placed on the tissue of the ridge, or even slightly above it, experience has shown that the tissue will, in time, hypertrophy and will not only come into contact with the underside of the bar but extend up along the sides of the bar into any space not occupied with the clip. Perhaps the best position of the bar in relation to the tissue is just high enough off the tissue to allow the tip of a mini proxy brush

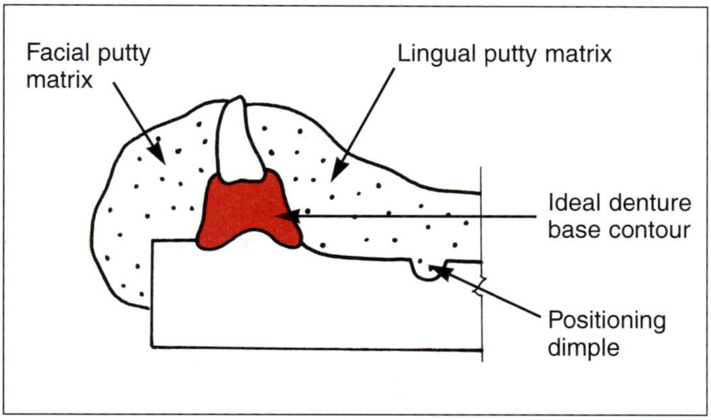

Fig 10-11 Putty matrix over patient-approved set-up and wax-up.

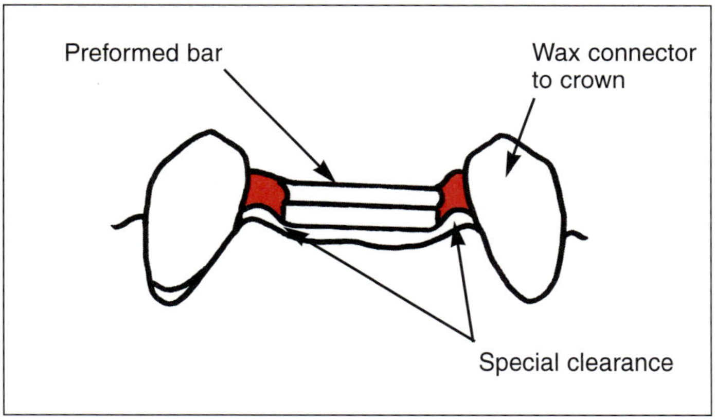

Fig 10-12 Relationship of plastic bar pattern to gingiva.

to pass under the bar. The patient must assume responsibility for daily stimulation of the tissue as well as keeping the undersurface free from plaque. The contours of the bar where it connects to the crowns or copings must also be carefully evaluated, as the clearance required for the marginal gingival tissue is even more critical than for the bar as a whole (Fig 10-12). The level of the bar in these areas will, almost without exception, need to be raised. In practical terms, this means that the bar must be cut short of the connector area, maintaining sufficient length for the clip, and then waxed into contact with the crown, usually in a curved segment. As this connector is closer to the incisal/occlusal plane, space may become a problem, even if there was adequate clearance over the straight length of the bar.

Usually the plastic bar pattern is cast to one side of the fixed component and soldered to the other side after relating the segments in the mouth or from the master cast. The preformed bar is soldered in similar fashion, usually with post solder after any ceramic component has been completed. The solder joints must always be larger in circumference than the bar itself. In the finishing and polishing of the bar, care must be taken not to touch the section of the bar that will receive the clip, since

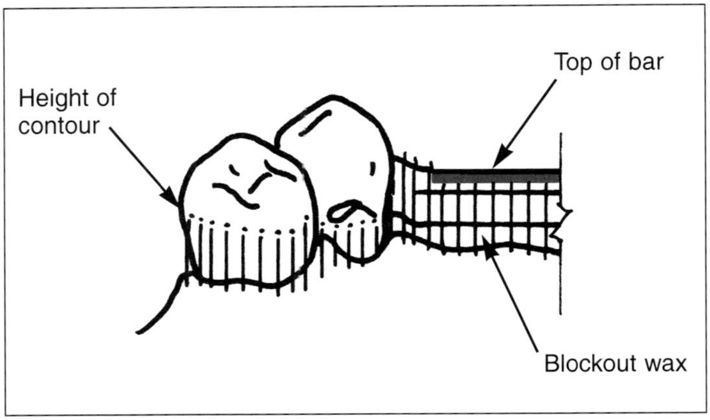

Fig 10-13 Blockout of bar and abutment crowns.

any change in dimension will reduce the retentive effect of the clip. Other areas of the bar—solder joints and tissue surface, for example—will receive the same degree of finish as the fixed units. When the fixed components including the bar have been completely assembled and finished, they are picked up in the final impression for the removable framework as described earlier so that they are available to the laboratory technician during the subsequent construction phases. To facilitate the removal of the impression from the cast, the space beneath the bar must be blocked out in the mouth. This step is easily accomplished by adapting a thin rope of soft utility wax to the underside of the bar before placing it in the mouth. The soft wax will adapt to the tissue, and any excess can be quickly removed with a hand instrument before the impression. This procedure will be far easier than trying to pack wax under the bar in the wet field of the mouth.

It is not essential to use the clip with the bar. In fact, in instances where space is at a real premium, the bar makes an ideal anterior rest for the partial. Conventional clasping or other attachment systems elsewhere in the mouth will then provide the necessary retention. This approach also serves as a less expensive alternative to fixed pontics in many situations, most commonly when mandibular incisors are missing and the option is either to include them with the fixed component as pontics or to replace them with the partial denture. As a result of adding the bar in the anterior region, the two sides are more effectively splinted and an ideal rest is created. A disadvantage to this use of the bar is that the patient is forced to wear the partial denture at all times for esthetic reasons.

Whether the clip will be used or not, the bar is to be blocked out along with the other components of the remaining dental arch. The superior surface of the bar is left free of blockout wax so that the partial denture casting will contact the bar along that surface up to the solder joint area, where a slight amount of relief is appropriate (Fig 10-13). This blockout of the bar presupposes that the bar and associated fixed components have been picked up from the mouth in their finished state and are a part

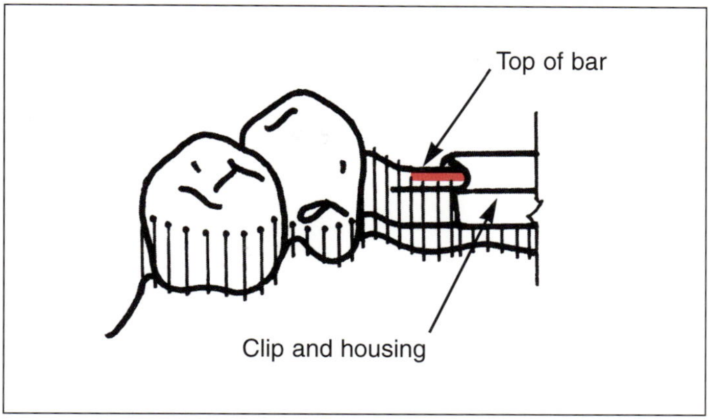

Fig 10-14 Blockout of bar and clip.

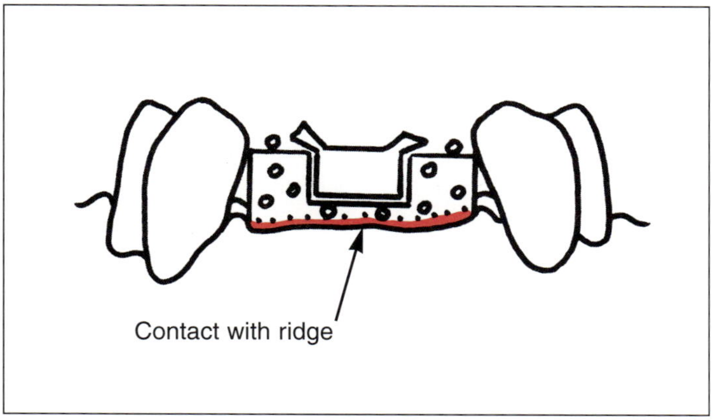

Fig 10-15 RPD casting–gold clip relationship before pick-up.

of the master cast submitted to the laboratory for construction of the framework. If a clip is to be used, it, along with its housing, must be in place on the bar at the time of blockout so that a refractory replica the exact size of the housing will be created (Fig 10-14). The clip must be placed in such a way as to ensure that its midline is parallel to the path of insertion, as indicated by the prepared guiding planes on the abutment teeth, permitting both wings of the clip to be flexed the same amount when the clip is activated during insertion and removal. The clip will be reproduced in the refractory cast to create an opening in the casting exactly where the clip is to be positioned. The outer surface of the casting adjacent to the opening will require retentive beads or loops to retain the attaching resin (Fig 10-15). The tooth-replacement retention in the area of any bar-clip attachment or the bar alone is to be metal with beads or other mechanical projections. This will always be superior to having that area only in resin, since the limited space will require the strength of the full metal coverage. The metal coverage must extend to the crest of the remaining ridge just anterior to the bar, with the remainder of the denture base in resin of the appropriate color. When that resin is thin, it will be necessary to have the laboratory opaque the facial aspect of the metal so that it will not be seen through the partially translucent denture base.

When the casting is returned from the laboratory, all components are seated in the mouth if some natural teeth are present, or on the master cast if all contacts are on fixed units, and its fit is corrected as required. If the casting contacts only the fixed components present on the master cast, either the clip or the clip housing, depending on the system in use, should be attached to the frame on the master cast with a small amount of autopolymerizing resin, either pink or tooth-colored, depending on the area of attachment. When the casting contacts teeth not associated with the fixed restorations present on the master cast as well as the fixed components, the clip should be attached in the mouth, with all components completely seated. Only after the clip is attached to the framework is the altered cast impression made (where indicated) and jaw relation records taken. The object is to have the framework and associated abutments in their final relationship before any support of the soft tissue is obtained. This will ensure that no misalignment occurs during processing of the denture bases.

Before the flasking of the denture bases, the fixed components are removed from the master cast so they will not be subjected to the high pressures of trial packing. The metal housing in the area of the clip is filled with a silicone mold release material or a putty to protect the clip and housing. The fully waxed denture is seated on the master cast, and the borders are sealed. The first half of the flasking will cover the resin cores that once supported the fixed components, in addition to any exposed areas of the framework, in the standard fashion. The silicone will make the clean-up of the clip area very easy because no stone will be present.

The clips, either metal or plastic, will eventually wear and will need replacement. In general, the plastic clips will wear much faster than the metal clips but, since they are now in a metal housing, they can be replaced in seconds at low cost. Their life expectancy can be improved in two very important ways. First, if the remaining teeth/fixed units are milled to 90 degrees to the path of insertion/removal, the wings of the clip will flex equally and minimally as the clip is activated. Second, if the patient can be made to take some responsibility for the method of insertion of the precision attachment partial (ie, never bite the partial to place but use only finger pressure), the load on the clip will be controlled. These two suggestions are applicable to all partial dentures but are especially pertinent to the precision attachment with a resilient component.

In replacing the plastic clip, any dental hand instrument that can fit inside the metal housing can be used to slide the old clip out of the housing. The new clip is placed on the insertion tool that is specific to that clip and snapped into place. Replacement of the metal clip will require that the old clip be ground out of the partial by making an access hole over the clip, usually just lingual to the replacement teeth. The hole must be large enough to allow access to the entire clip and its retentive extensions. These retentive extensions are covered with a thin coat of autopolymerizing resin of the appropriate color. If the coating resin is a fibered repair resin, the fibers are removed by sifting them out through a 2 × 2 gauze. The resin

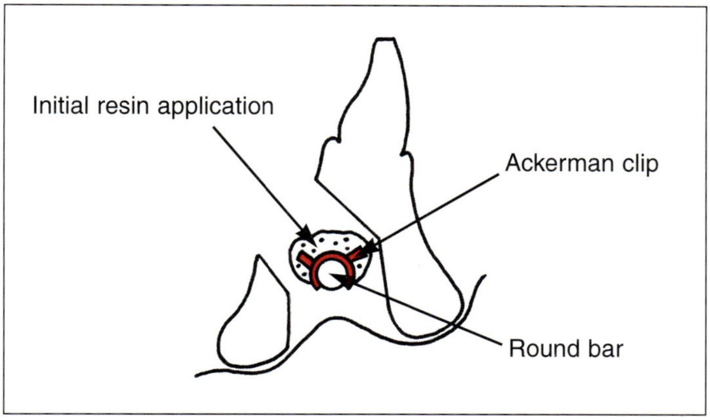

Fig 10-16 Cross section of mandibular overdenture showing replacement of Ackerman clip (gold).

should be placed on the clip as quickly as possible and the clip placed in the pressure pot to cure. Once the resin is hard, any excess can be removed and the clip placed on the bar, making sure that it is aligned with the path of insertion and the partial is seated over the clip. By completely covering the retentive elements of the clip with resin outside the mouth, the clinician will ensure that no voids are created when the clip is actually connected to the partial in the mouth. Only enough additional resin need be added by picking up polymer with a wetted brush and placing it through the access hole to create a solid joint (Fig 10-16). The patient is instructed to close lightly into maximum occlusion to verify the proper base-clip relationship and then open the mouth slightly while the clinician holds the denture in place. Once the layer of resin has completely cured in the mouth, the partial is carefully removed and the remainder of the required resin added to fill the internal contour to its pre-repair condition. The exterior hole is filled to excess, after which the partial is placed in the pressure pot for the entire curing time. By filling to excess and then finishing away the excess, the density of the added resin will be maximized.

The bar-clip combination offers a relatively inexpensive attachment system that has been used successfully for a few generations. It is adaptable to many situations and easy to maintain. Its only real disadvantage is that it does require a good deal of space, both vertically and horizontally, and so cannot be used universally.

Intracoronal Precision Attachments

The intracoronal attachment that is classified as precision comes from the manufacturer as two components: a matrix and a patrix. These are often accompanied by a paralleling guide that fits into the dental surveyor as well as devices to activate the attachment after fabrication. The matrix is waxed into the crown or bonded into a preparation in the tooth. The patrix is attached to the framework in some fashion, usually by soldering. In many instances, the patrix will have some retentive component that can be activated and readjusted as wear occurs.

These attachments, being machined to close tolerances (0.001 inch on the average), cannot be expected to allow for controlled freedom in rotation of a denture base and, as a result, are used in all tooth or tooth/implant-supported partial dentures. There are a number of intracoronal attachments that have an integral hinged component intended to offer stress relief to a distal extension base. The use of this hinged attachment does not, in my opinion, fulfill the need to distribute the maximum load to the selected abutments. Instead, it places an uncontrolled amount of force on the tissue least likely to withstand the load, the edentulous ridge tissues. Since we know that resorption of the edentulous ridge is an ongoing, generally irreversible process, the use of any hinged device places an additional maintenance requirement on the clinician. The distal extension base must be kept in ideal contact with the underlying tissues through relines to minimize soft tissue impingement and stripping of tissue. I see no need for this type of attachment in the modern partial denture.

The standard intracoronal attachments that contain no moving parts do, however, offer excellent retention and esthetics for the tooth-borne partial. Since these attachment systems become a part of the crown or pontic, they must be contained within the normal contours of these restorations. The average dimension of the intracoronal attachment is just over 1.5 mm and, allowing for a minimum of 0.5 mm of metal in the crown internal to the matrix, it can be easily seen that a minimum of 2 mm of reduction in the area of the attachment is essential to keep the final unit within normal contours. It may be that bonding the patrix into a prepared cavity in the tooth would require less axial reduction than for a casting, but this treatment modality is in its infancy without longitudinal studies to support its use.

There is general agreement that, in addition to the axial space requirements, the tooth must have sufficient clinical crown length to accept a matrix with a minimum vertical height of 3.5 mm. The length of most matrices as received from the manufacturer is 6 mm, but it is not common to find a crown capable of accepting the total length. Obviously, the greater vertical length of the attachment complex, the greater the potential retention and stability that can be expected. There are a number of split attachments that have some form of latch (Sterngold GL, for example). This can be effective in shorter vertical lengths, since the actual retentive mechanism is a split casting with a ridge at its most gingival portion (a minimum of 2.62 mm is required for the GL) (Fig 10-17). Because of the split casting, the ridge can compress on itself and snap into a recess in the matrix.

These space requirements must be taken into careful consideration during the diagnostic waxing and positioning of the denture teeth. In the younger patient, where large pulp chambers and a lack of secondary dentin are found, it may not be possible to use an intracoronal attachment (extracoronal attachments will be necessary for these patients). The width of the matrix in a buccolingual direction will be in the range of 3 mm, a dimension that can be accommodated in most abutment teeth. For

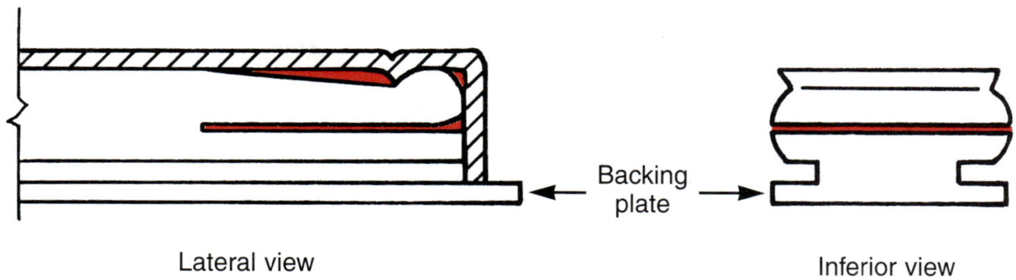

Fig 10-17 Intracoronal attachment (Sterngold GL gingival latch). Red denotes space within attachment latch area.

example, the width of the patrix for the Sterngold GL is either 2.43 mm for the standard head or 1.77 mm for the micro head.

Before mouth preparation on the actual abutment teeth, all guiding plane preparations on the remaining teeth that will not be treated with crowns or other castings must be made and verified. Making the attachments and any guiding planes on their crowns to match the path of insertion/removal as it exists on the other prepared teeth is more practical than making the attachment containing crowns first and then trying to parallel guiding planes to match the path. Since these attachments are very precise, it is nearly impossible to match their path after they are in place. The same system of diagnostic mouth preparation as suggested for the conventional partial denture must be employed with a careful verification of the check cast before beginning the actual preparation of the teeth to be crowned.

It should be obvious that any master cast for the construction of the crowns must include all other teeth involved with the partial denture. The clinician must determine the desired path of insertion/removal and transfer this spatial relationship to the technician through the use of three widely separated tripod marks, placed with the vertical arm of the surveyor in a locked position.

Laboratory construction of intracoronal precision attachment crown and pontic units is not difficult, although some experience is necessary to use the surveyor and special tools to position the matrices perfectly parallel to the indicated path of insertion. Some discussion with the technician is needed as to the extent of the porcelain coverage on the abutment crowns, since the matrix will require a small amount (0.4 mm minimum) of metal around it that is free of porcelain (Fig 10-18). These abutments will often also require milled guiding planes and appropriate contours to accept rests, all of which will influence the cutback of the metal for veneering.

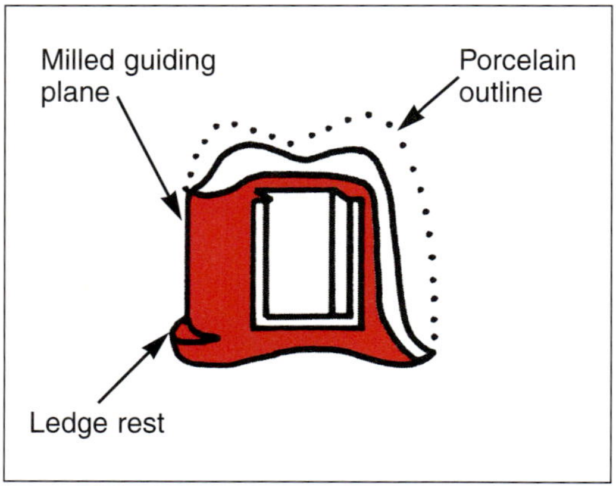

Fig 10-18 Veneer outline for intracoronal attachment.

The intracoronal attachment will not normally be indicated on the mesial surface of anterior teeth because the alteration of contour will, most likely, prove to be unacceptable (the canines being the only possible exception). Generally speaking, anterior edentulous spaces are better filled with fixed pontics than with components of the removable partial.

When the crowns have been completed and have been found to be acceptable for esthetics and occlusion, the final impression for the removable framework is made. A firm-setting elastomeric impression material is used, either silicone or polyether, in a custom tray with ample retention (holes and adhesive) to ensure that the impression material does not separate from the tray during removal of the impression from the mouth. These materials are not intended to impress large undercuts, as may be found on unprepared natural teeth. Since the goal of the final impression is to relate the fixed components to the remainder of the arch and to allow the pick-up of these components without distorting the final impression, it is often necessary to block out large undercuts, furcations, undersurfaces of pontics, and any other area where the resistance to removal is apt to be so high as to threaten the integrity of the final impression. Any number of materials can be used for the blockout of these unusable areas; wax, temporary cement, cotton pellets, and alginate are examples that should be considered.

Ideally, the crowns and other fixed components should come out in the impression; repositioning them in the impression does not guarantee accuracy. As discussed earlier, resin dies should be available to insert in the crowns prior to pouring the master cast. The modern impression materials used in these situations can be comfortably transported to the dental laboratory without fear of distortion and the construction of the master cast left to the technician. A diagnostic cast must accompany the final impression to inform the technician of the prescribed design of the framework. It is usually necessary to make an alginate duplication of the master cast containing the fixed components in order to obtain a diagnostic cast, since the master impression may require a burning of the tray to recover it. It is much easier to convey specific requirements via a diagnostic cast with a neat and careful drawing of the outline of the framework than to try to describe the desired outcome over the phone or on the work authorization form.

The same requirements of design and construction as described for the conventional partial denture must be adhered to for the precision attachment framework. When the frame and master cast are returned to the clinician, the fit of the frame in the mouth and to the crowns must be verified before the patrices are picked up in resin, either in the mouth or on the master cast. The decision as to where best to join the attachments to the framework is dependent on many factors and there is no one correct way. It must be remembered, however, that in every instance the frame/attachment relationship must be identical from the mouth to the master cast before the construction can continue. Most intracoronal attachments will be joined to the framework by soldering because space is likely to be a critical factor.

The fit of the framework must be reverified after the soldering operation in every instance. Only when the tooth/frame relation meets the highest standards can other procedures be undertaken, ie, altered cast impressions and jaw relation records. The completion of the case, once these steps are done, is relatively standard as far as positioning of the denture teeth and waxing, processing, and finishing of the base are concerned. An area of special consideration is the protection of the patrix connection when the amount of resin over or around this area is minimal (less than 2 mm of tooth structure or base resin). In these instances, metal occlusal surfaces are to be constructed, usually in type IV gold, and added to the denture teeth to ensure that subsequent wear will not break through to the patrix.

At insertion of the intracoronal attachment partial denture, any undercuts to the path of insertion/removal will have to be carefully identified and recontoured to fully seat the partial. Since the path of insertion will be so precise, the finished partial must never be forced to place on initial seating until all possible undercuts in resin have been identified and adjusted. The soft tissues of the mouth occlusal to areas of slight undercut may compress and allow the full seating of the partial but will not allow the partial to be removed without pain or discomfort to the patient, sometimes with great difficulty. If pressure-indicating paste is placed on all resin areas and the partial is inserted with light pressure until resistance is felt, either by the clinician or by the patient, areas of potential difficulty can be identified without fear of tissue irritation.

There remains only the activation of the attachment, in those attachment systems where this possibility exists. In general, patients should be informed of the intention to use only the lightest activation that will satisfy their needs for retention, since the lower the level of activation, the better the chance to reduce distortion and the need for repeated adjustments. Activation is accomplished with the use of specific tools, provided by the manufacturer, which distort the patrix by increasing the opening of the split areas of the metal (Fig 10-19). The tools are carefully calibrated to ensure that overactivation does not occur, a frightening situation where the partial denture cannot be removed from the mouth without excessive force. For this reason it is not wise to allow patients to reactivate their attachments by themselves. Assuming that every aspect of construction of the intracoronal precision attachment partial has been done to the highest standards, the attachments should need only periodic reactivation, undertaken as a part of normal recall activities. Systematic recall for these patients is perhaps as critical as high standards of construction for the long-term success of the entire treatment. Certainly, these two components of treatment are far more important than variations in design of the partial denture.

A wide assortment of intracoronal attachments is available to the clinician, all

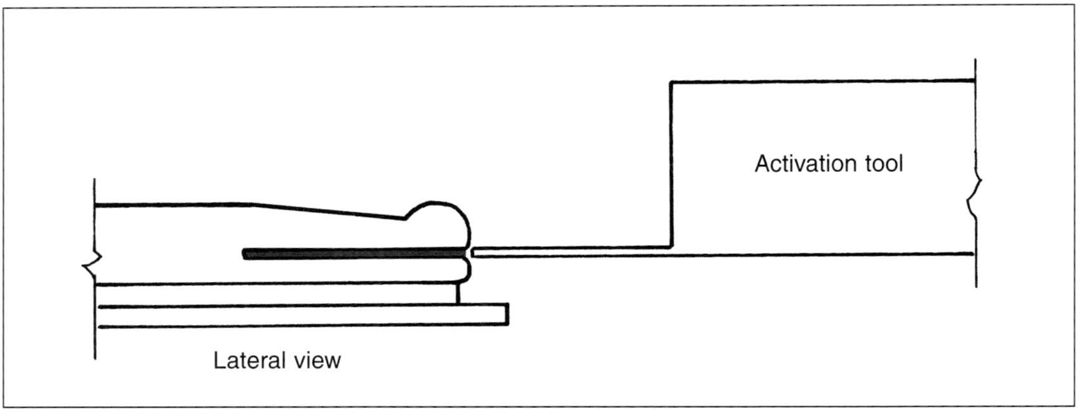

Fig 10-19 Reactivation of Sterngold GL attachment.

based on the same general principles described here. Dental technicians will have their favorites, depending on their experience; however, their experience is based on fabrication issues and not on clinical evaluation. Therefore, while one attachment system may be easier to construct, it does not follow that the system will work as well as some other type over the expected lifespan of 20± years. The sheer number of attachments precludes that any one clinician or technician will have had sufficient experience working with all attachments to define the selection in any scientific manner. (See listing of attachment manuals and manufacturers at the end of this chapter).

Intracoronal Semiprecision Attachments

Because of the very low tolerances of the precision attachment, little stress relief is possible when it is used on Class I partial dentures, especially in the mandible. When only a few compromised mandibular anterior teeth are available as abutments, as is so often the case, many clinicians elect to relieve the stress of mastication to the abutments by splinting all remaining teeth and transferring some of the load to the edentulous ridge. While it is theoretically possible to do that with precision attachments that utilize a moving component in the patrix, as stated earlier this is not advisable. There is a type of attachment, usually referred to as a semiprecision rest attachment, that utilizes an intracoronal box and a resilient lingual clasp arm, preferably wrought, for the actual retention. The bottom of the box in the crown has a slight lip and a rounded base that allows the patrix rest to rotate slightly in function but that will not, because of the lip, slip distally and unseat (Fig 10-20). To disengage, the entire partial must move vertically the distance of the raised lip before the patrix is free of the matrix. The esthetic effect of the semiprecision attachment is exactly the same as for the precision intracoronal attachment: no evidence of the partial denture on the facial aspect of the abutments.

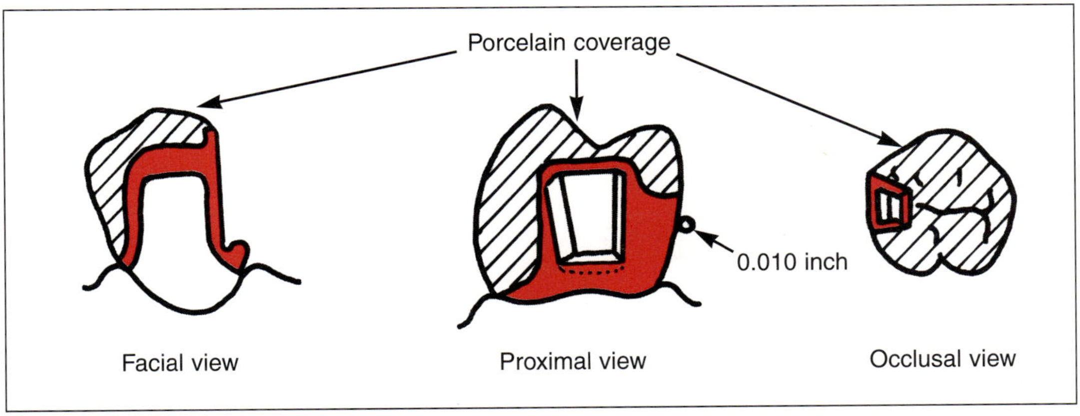

Fig 10-20 Cross sections of semiprecision intracoronal attachment, Thompson dowel rest.

The Thompson dowel attachment is the best known of this type of device. It is made by waxing the matrix to a homemade former and then creating the patrix rest pattern in resin directly in the finished casting of the abutment. Similar attachment forms are made by some commercial manufacturers (Preat N-L attachment, for example).

The semiprecision attachment, almost always created in the dental laboratory either in wax or by milling the completed casting, can be used with a lingual retentive clasp arm in Class II, III, and IV situations as well as in the bilateral distal extension situation. However, their use is not as easy to defend because the space they require in the crown will be the same as the precision attachment, without the retentive effect found in most precision patrices. If a posterior isolated abutment on a tooth-borne side of the partial is less than ideal and without a projected lifespan expected of the partial, the Thompson dowel attachment is indicated for the more anterior abutment tooth (usually a premolar). When the distal abutment tooth is lost, the partial can be quickly converted to a distal extension (either Class I or II) without having to be concerned about the stress relief of the attachment system.

A matrix former can be easily handmade in wax, attached to a straight resin sprue of sufficient length and dimension to allow it to be placed in the vertical arm of the dental surveyor, and cast in any alloy (usually a nonprecious partial denture alloy). It is finished and polished and then machined using the side of a large, flat disk to ensure that the walls of the matrix will have no undercut areas. The original Thompson dowel attachment had both a right and a left matrix former, the lingual walls of which were set at right angles to the internal wall. The buccal walls diverged slightly to allow ease of rotation while still providing a guiding plane surface parallel to the path of insertion/removal. The buccal divergence also allows easier placement of the attachment for insertion by the patient. The metal former is lubricated with a silicone spray, and wax is added in excess to create the matrix. The wax pattern is removed from the ma-

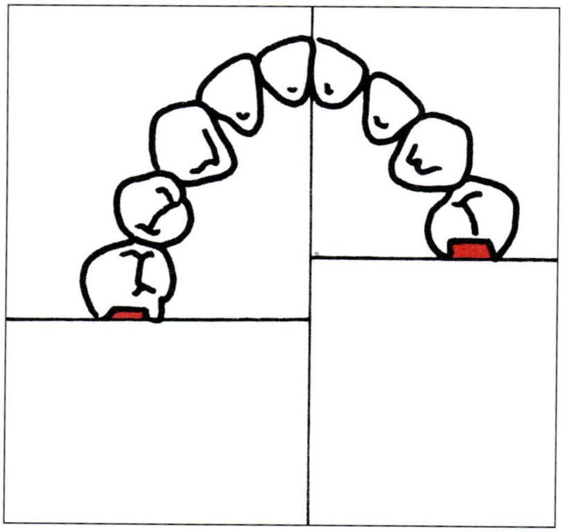

Fig 10-21 Parallel placement of Thompson dowel rest.

trix former and reduced to have walls approximately 0.3 mm thick. The crown pattern is cut away on the distal aspect to a thickness of 0.3 mm and the matrix pattern is added to the crown using the surveyor to carry the wax matrix to place. Once the matrix has been fully tacked into place and the contours reestablished, the former is removed from the wax pattern.

Since this attachment is semiprecision, it can be completely hand waxed without the use of the matrix former. Tapered burs are used in the wax pattern to create the walls to the same dimensions and angles. A round bur can be used to create the depression for the rotational ridge. When shaping wax with a bur, it is obvious that a very slow speed must be used. For this reason, a belt-driven, low-speed and high-torque handpiece is often used. The sophisticated milling machines commonly found in laboratories that specialize in this type of prosthodontic work have specially made wax-cutting burs that, when used in combination with precise speed control, make the shaping of the matrix a relatively simple procedure.

It should be obvious that the matrix form must be set parallel to the path of insertion/removal as dictated by the guiding planes prepared on any nonrestored teeth present in the arch that will be used as abutments. When this attachment is used for a Class I partial denture, the internal walls of the matrix must be set parallel to each other and at right angles to the midsagittal plane of the arch (Fig 10-21). This positioning of the matrices is essential to allow rotation of the bilateral distal extension bases. When the terminal abutment is a canine, it is often necessary to shape the distal half of the tooth like a premolar to place the distal surface parallel to the distal surface on the opposite side of the arch (Fig 10-22). When the remaining teeth are to be splinted, as they often are in these cases, a premolar can be cantilevered off the terminal canine to contain the attachment. Since the actual retention of the partial will be created using a lingual wire circumferential clasp, the use of the premolar pontic will allow a longer clasp arm than would be possible on the canine, with a more natural approach to a mesiolingual undercut area (Fig 10-23). If the abutment teeth are not to be splinted across the arch, double abutting must be considered, with additional rests and guiding planes prepared on the nonsplinted teeth. The use of this attachment in a nonsplinted mandibular first premolar, for example, would be contraindicated due to the possible load that could be placed on the tooth if the distal extension base were not kept in full con-

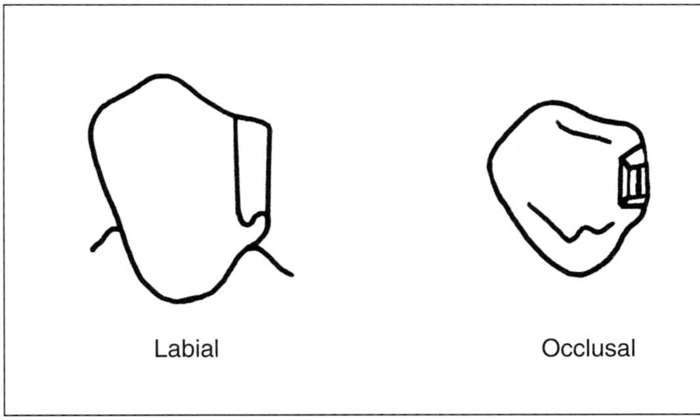

Fig 10-22 Alteration of contour (canine) to accommodate precision attachment.

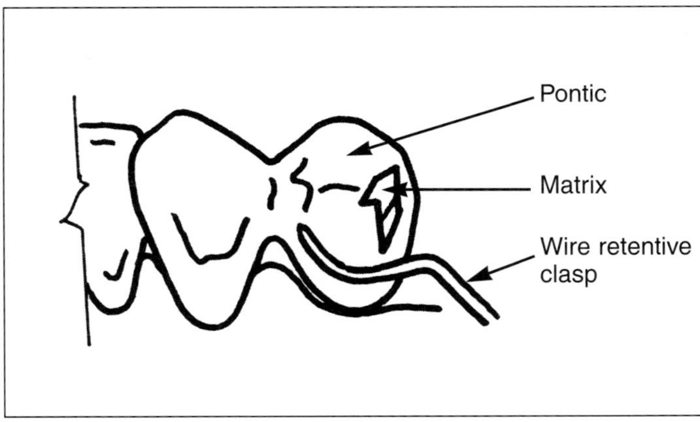

Fig 10-23 Cantilevered first premolar to contain attachment (Thompson dowel).

tact and support through the original altered cast impression and subsequent relines.

The lingual surface of the waxed crown(s) is prepared to accept the terminal third of a light wire (20 gauge) circumferential clasp running to the mesiolingual. The entire lingual surface can be shaped to allow the clasp arm to lie in a depression in the metal, with the final one third passing into a 0.010-inch undercut relative to the path of insertion/removal of the matrix and the remainder of the guiding planes in the mouth. The clasp arm is to be extended as far to the mesial as the embrasure contour will allow to create the longest possible retentive arm (Fig 10-24). The height of contour must be planned to leave a 1-mm space between the gingival border of the clasp and the gingival tissue.

Once the castings have been completed and veneered, they are picked up from the mouth in the final impression for the partial denture. The patrices are now formed in resin and their tangs in either resin or wax. At this time, a decision on the method of attachment of the patrices to the framework will have to be made. If the patrices are to be soldered to the framework, the area of attachment should be all in metal with the

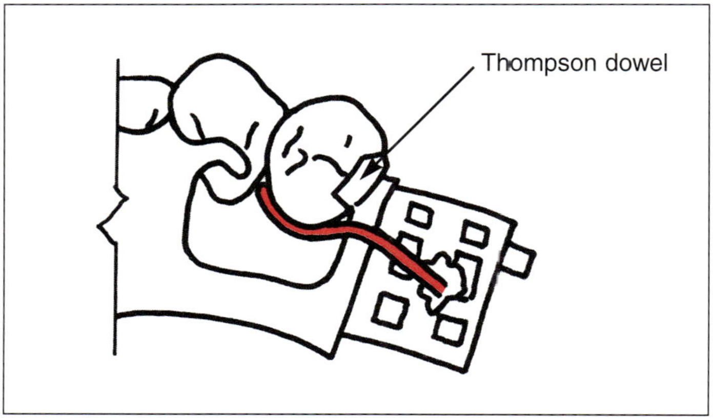

Fig 10-24 Lingual retentive wire with full extension into embrasure.

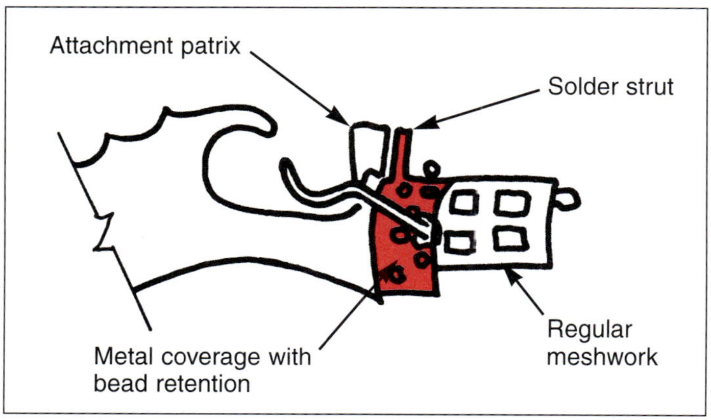

Fig 10-25 Metal coverage of ridge under soldered attachment.

internal finishing line distal to the solder area (Fig 10-25). This would require that the relief wax be placed distal to the soldering area. If the intent is to attach the patrices to the frame with resin and keep them in resin, then an evaluation of the available space occlusal to the meshwork must be made. Remember, when space is at a premium, the soldering method of attachment is preferred. With adequate space, there is an advantage to keeping the connection in resin so that the attachment component can be replaced with minimum destruction to the partial.

When the shape of the tang is established, the wax and resin pattern is invested and cast in the same alloy or one slightly softer than was used for the crown. This is done so any wear with time will occur on the patrix, which are relatively easy to replace, rather than on the matrices. Type III gold will probably be slightly softer than the ceramic alloy chosen for the crowns. The master cast, with the patrices in place, is now ready for blockout and duplication. The waxing of the framework will depend on the manner in which the patrices are to be attached.

Once again, the framework is protected from any internal finishing by the technician and, only after a quality fit is verified in the mouth, will the patrices be attached to the frame, either on the cast or in the mouth. Care must be taken to ensure that the patrices are fully contacting the internal wall of the matrix when they are added to the frame, since it is in this relationship that the altered cast impression must be made. Now the altered cast impressions are made, even though the clasp arms have not yet been added to the casting. The altered cast with its jaw relation record is returned to the laboratory for the addition of the wire clasp arms and completion of the case.

Since there is no labiobuccal clasp arm on this type of partial denture, a Class V cavity is cut into the most anterior denture tooth to serve as a ledge where the patient can place a fingernail to remove the partial. The Thompson dowel attachment offers freedom to rotate for the Class I partial denture, with ease of adjustment of the wire retentive clasp. The only disadvantage to this type of attachment is the bulk of the matrix and the need for 3.5 mm of vertical height.

Extracoronal Attachments

There are a variety of extracoronal attachments available to the clinician. Some of these are rigid; that is, they do not allow any rotation of the partial in function. Others are hinged, offering a stress-breaking action to the distal extension base. More recently, a number of resilient extracoronal attachments have come on the market that permit a limited amount of movement of the denture base for the Class I partial situation. Both the rigid and the resilient attachments have a distinct place in the tooth- and tissue-borne partial denture. The need for hinged attachments is less obvious; the rationale for their use can be questioned if one recognizes the need to utilize the remaining possible abutment teeth for maximum support and retention and to reduce the load on the soft tissues as much as possible. The conventional distal extension removable partial denture creates stress relief through rest placement, light clasping, altered cast impressions, and careful maintenance, with periodic relines to keep the base movement to a minimum. If the conventional partial denture, constructed to these principles, is potentially as successful as longitudinal studies would have us believe, there seems little advantage to placing greater load on the extension base through the use of hinged attachments. It has been my experience that the hinged attachment has great potential to become destructive to the soft tissue unless it is very carefully maintained and replaced as soon as it begins to show lateral movement in addition to its planned vertical rotation. For that reason, I do not consider its use justifiable.

The great advantage of the extracoronal attachment is that it does not alter the normal contour of the abutment crown, being entirely outside of these contours. An additional advantage of the rigid attachment is that the entire length of the attachment, from the gingival tissue to the occlusal plane, can be used for retention, making it invaluable in situations in which the abutment teeth are short.

A simple rigid extracoronal attachment is one commonly referred to as the *pin-tube attachment* (Fig 10-26). For most of these, the pin (patrix) is added to the fixed unit and the matrix (tube) to the partial denture. The attachments can easily be made by hand. They are also available from attachment manufacturers (Preci-Vertex from Preat Corp, Interlock and Tubelock

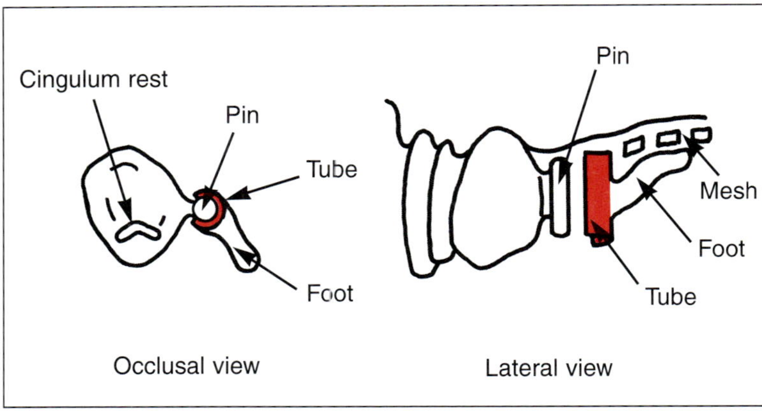

Fig 10-26 Pin-tube attachment.

from APM Sterngold, for example). Some intracoronal pin and tube attachments can be used as extracoronal attachments by reversing the patrix and matrix so that, instead of having the matrix in the crown, it becomes part of the partial denture (cylindrical slide CM attachment from American Precision Metals). Recently, resilient retentive sleeves have been added to the matrices of pin-tube attachments. The most commonly used of this special form is the vertical Hader bar. A similar current form is the Preci-Vertix from Preat Corp, which, according to the manufacturer's claims, can be used either as a rigid attachment or, reducing by 0.3 to 0.5 mm the coronal portion of the patrix, as a resilient attachment. All of these simple attachments can be constructed using the same principles with little expected variation. They differ from the older systems in that the matrix is lined with a resilient material that can be easily and inexpensively replaced as needed for retention. The matrices come with a precisely machined metal cover that has retentive contours on its outer surface to which resin can adhere. The metal matrix covers are intended to stay in the partial for its normal life, allowing the resilient inner matrices to be replaced.

A slightly different attachment system that is well-known and has been used for more than 30 years is the Ceka attachment (Ceka NV, Antwerp, Belgium). This attachment differs from the others in that the patrix is a split metal post that is adjustable and snaps into a metal matrix attached to the proximal surface of the abutment crown. This system has many modifications for use in a variety of situations. The patrix post is threaded so that it can be screwed into the holding device and easily replaced if damaged or worn. A spacer ring is used to allow the possibility of stress relief, creating a vertical space of 0.3 mm when the spacer has been removed after construction. This space allows a small amount of rotation of the partial denture, which will place some of the load on the tissues of the denture base. A recent Ceka innovation is called the

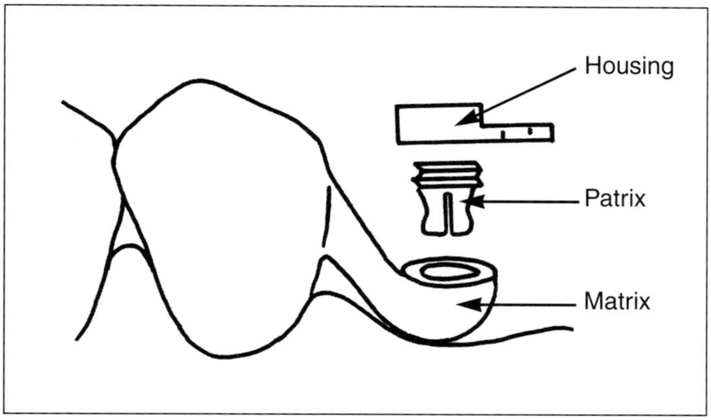

Fig 10-27 Ceka Revax attachment.

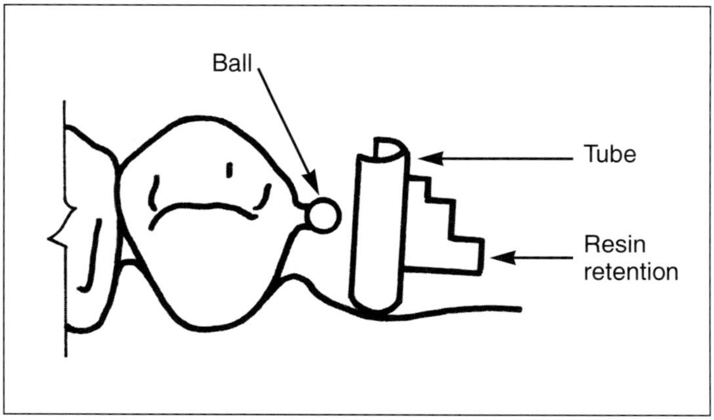

Fig 10-28 Roach attachment (ball and tube).

Ceka Revax attachment. This system places the matrix in contact with the gingival tissues in a way that allows easy access for hygiene, both under the matrix and between the matrix and the axial surface of the abutment crown, so that the gingival tissues are never compromised (Fig 10-27).

A very old system that has been in use since the turn of the century is the Roach attachment. The patrix of this attachment is a partially split, adjustable round ball that extends from the axial surface of the abutment crown. The ball comes as a finished casting that can be soldered to the axial surface of a crown or cast to. The matrix of this system is a tube, in much the same form as discussed previously. In its earliest form, the tube was made from plate gold and was attached to the partial denture by means of a metal tang that had been soldered to the tube. The modern edition has a tube with one form to be used if the attachment is to be soldered to the framework, another if the matrix is to be attached with resin (Fig 10-28).

Since the patrix is a round ball, the contact with the matrix is only at the circumference, which allows for more rotation than any of the other systems. The increased stress relief available with this sys-

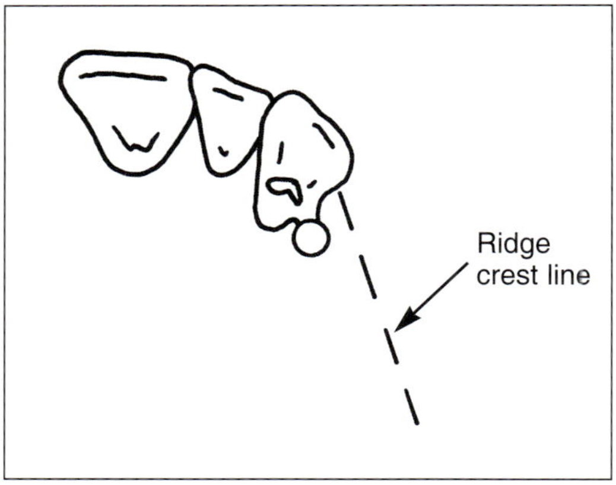

Fig 10-29 Extracoronal attachment placed lingual to ridge crest.

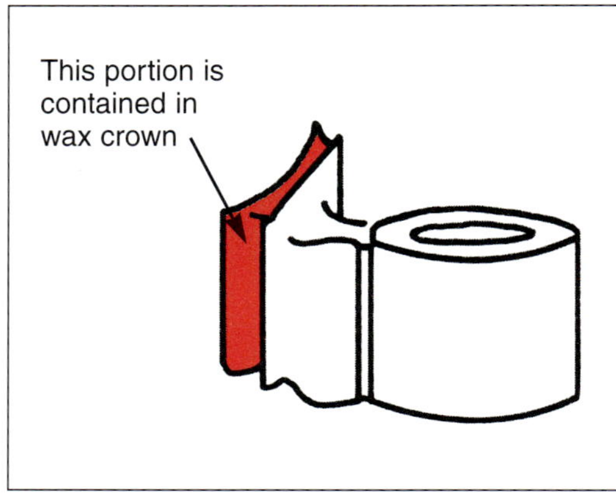

Fig 10-30 ERA patrix, castable plastic.

tem indicates its use in compromised dentitions for which a conscious decision has been made to transfer load from the abutments to the supporting tissues of the denture bases. The exact amount of rotation allowed with the Roach attachment is a factor of the space between the tube and the axial wall, since the tube can only allow rotation to the point where it comes in contact with the crown. In all the systems that allow rotation, the amount of movement that is desired is slight; the use of the altered cast impression and the relines that are made, when indicated, keep the amount of space between the base and the tissues to a minimum. If the precision attachment partial denture is ignored for long periods of time, no attachment system will permit control of the rotational forces.

After all fixed units have been waxed to full contour and milled in wax for maximum guiding plane surfaces, the patrices, of whatever system has been chosen, are added to the axial surfaces of the abutment crowns using the special alignment tools provided by the manufacturer. The patrices are generally patterns, made in some form of hard resin that is amenable to burnout and casting in standard ceramo-metal alloys. The alignment tool is placed in the dental surveyor at the same tilt of master cast as was used for the wax milling of the guiding plane surfaces. It is critical that the path of insertion/removal to be used takes into account the height of contour of the edentulous soft tissues as well as the remaining teeth.

The plastic pattern, or preformed metal patrix, is to be placed somewhat lingual to the center of the proximal surface (Fig 10-29). This step ensures that the bulk of the matrix will not interfere with the esthetics of the buccal cusp of the replacement denture tooth. The average patient can tolerate a slight excess of contour to the lingual because esthetics are not involved. The patrix (in the pin systems) is to extend from a contact with the edentulous ridge just lingual to the crest of the ridge to the occlusal plane. This length can be maintained in systems that utilize an open tube. If the system requires a capped housing, the patrix will have to be shortened to accommodate the housing. The decision of which type of system to employ often hinges on the amount of vertical space available. The patrix pin must extend far enough out from the abutment tooth that floss or cotton yarn can be passed under the pin and up to the marginal gingiva. Most plastic patterns come with a self-limiting platform that, when waxed into the normal contour of the abutment tooth, automatically controls the extension into the edentulous area (Fig 10-30).

When the teeth bearing the extracoronal attachments are to be veneered with porcelain, resin, or composite, the extension of the cutback for the veneer is critical. The veneering material must not be allowed to contact the matrix portion of the attachment. In most cases, this requirement will cause the margin of metal to extend further to the facial and lingual surfaces than it would in a veneered crown not involved with the attachment. This extension beyond the normal cutback is generally in the area of 1.0 to 1.5 mm; esthetics is usually not a problem given that the attachment is most often on the distal proximal surface of the abutment tooth.

Fortunately for both clinician and technician, the manufacturers of attachments provide excellent instructional material, generally at no cost. Since systems are constantly being redesigned, the inclusion of great technical detail in any text is apt to be a waste of time.

After casting, the technician is careful to leave the patrices untouched; any finishing and polishing will decrease the retention of the system. The fixed units are finished and veneered and are then included on the master cast for the partial denture framework as described earlier. This step is essential for the extracoronal attachment because the patrices are so small they would not stand up if impressed and poured in stone. By having the actual casting on the master cast, the technician creating the partial denture can wax out the contours and prepare the refractory cast so that the attachment of the matrices is precise and accurate.

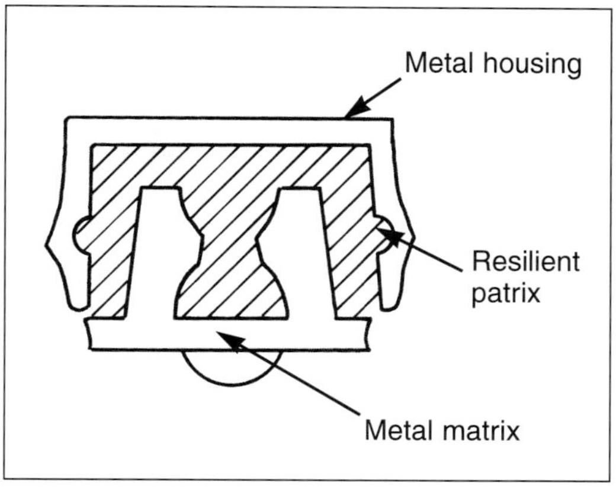

Fig 10-31 ERA cross section, overdenture matrix.

When all remaining teeth in the arch are part of the fixed component, the matrices are best picked up on the master cast and verified in the mouth. When some of the abutments are natural teeth not associated with the fixed units, the task of picking up the attachments becomes slightly more complex since the stone replicas of these abutments may be damaged. In this situation, it is best to place all the fixed components in the mouth, fit the frame, and then attach the matrices with autopolymerizing or light-activated resin. The complete assembly must then, of course, be returned to the master cast for verification. Tolerances for the relationship of components in the precision attachment partial denture are much finer than for the conventional partial, so the use of magnification whenever possible is essential.

Most of the extracoronal attachment systems are self-aligning when it comes to joining the matrices to the patrices. The components need only be fully seated on each other and the resin applied. Some systems—the Roach, for example—have aligning tools for the matrices that are to be used with the dental surveyor. These systems must be attached on the bench.

For each of these systems, the decision whether to solder the matrices to the framework or to attach them with resin must be made on an individual basis, with the space requirement being the biggest factor. Both means work well and, with care, will not cause problems.

The set-up and wax-up of the partial denture containing extracoronal attachments are generally not complicated except for placing the denture tooth that sits over the attachment assembly. Often, this first tooth will need to be hollowed out to a mere shell. To ensure that the denture base resin does not show through the tooth, it will be necessary to pack a small amount of tooth-colored resin, preferably heat-curing, under the tooth before the remainder of the denture base is packed. When space is at a premium, metal occlusal surfaces are the only way to prevent rapid wear and associated destruction of the attachment assembly. The cost of adding a small onlay or one-half crown form to the partial is minimal compared to the cost of repairing the attachment partial denture down the road.

For any or all of these systems, when used in a Class I or II arch, primarily in the mandible, an altered cast must be made *after* the attachments have been joined to the framework. A separate appointment will often be required to obtain this impression and the following jaw relation records, because the addition of resin to the matrices/patrices requires access to the retentive meshwork in the same areas as would be used to join the altered cast trays. With the attachments fully seated, the altered cast impression can be made with confidence since the support of both the hard and soft tissues has been optimized.

Resilient Attachments

A final classification of extracoronal attachments remains to be discussed. The use of resilient materials to line the matrices of some of the tube-type attachments has already been mentioned in passing. These could be classified as resilient attachments, but the term is more apt to be restricted to a relatively recent development, best illustrated by the ERA and O-SO attachment systems. Both of these systems were developed to allow for stress relief and for simple and rapid replacement of the resilient components. Both systems wear out quickly but are so easily replaced that some patients can do the job themselves.

The ERA system is similar to the Ceka attachment already described, the difference being that the patrix in the ERA is a plastic material that snaps into a matrix ring attached to the crown (Fig 10-31). The ring comes as a castable plastic pattern. Four different levels of retention are available with four slightly different plastic patrices. A metal housing with internal retentive grooves for the plastic inserts and external ridges for resin retention is included with the attachment system. The patrices are color-coded, with the white unit being the most flexible and progressing through orange to blue to gray as the most rigid. Recent studies have indicated that after a short time, there is no clinical difference between the three colored units. Most situ-

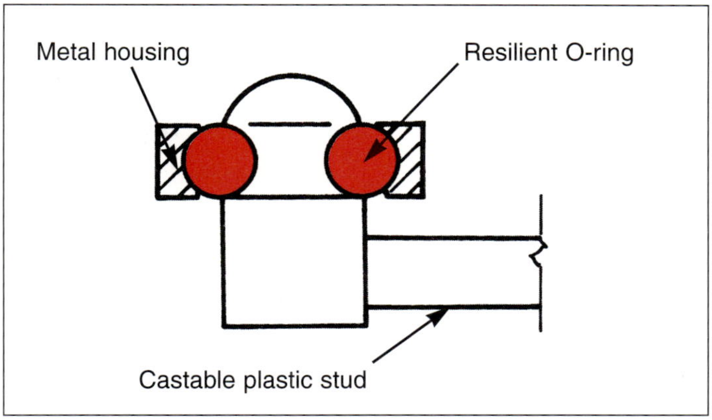

Fig 10-32 Resilient stud attachment (O-SO), extracoronal, in cross section.

ations will need only the white patrix, as the amount of retention it gives combined with other frictional retentive components of the partial denture, is more than adequate. A trephine bur that allows rapid removal of the worn patrix is provided. Also provided is an insertion tool that carries the new patrix into the partial and forces it to place in the housing. The entire operation takes less than a minute. A processing patrix is also a part of the system. It allows some space for movement of the patrix in the housing to create stress relief, as it is slightly longer than the colored units that are installed after processing. The ERA has become very popular due to its ease of replacement and the slight amount of flexibility it allows.

The O-SO attachment is actually classified as a stud attachment, with a patrix that looks somewhat like a doorknob and with a rubber O-ring matrix. The O-ring comes, in its most recent form, with a metal housing not unlike that used with other systems (Fig 10-32). The system also uses a processing ring that is replaced by a soft rubber ring before being placed in the patient's mouth. The ring is quite soft and therefore quickly worn, but it can be easily replaced. The old ring can be picked out with an explorer or small tweezers and the new ring pushed into place with any small blunt-ended instrument. The patrix comes as a castable plastic pattern that can be attached as an extracoronal attachment or, in a slightly different form, as an overdenture stud. Implant manufacturers provide a similar stud and O-ring attachments that screw directly into the fixture or onto the transmucosal abutment. It is the most flexible of all the attachment systems and is therefore of greatest use in situations where tooth support is minimal.

For the most part, the metal housings for the matrices of the ERA, the O-SO, and other resilient systems will be attached to the framework of the removable partial denture with resin, not soldered. These matrices can be related in the mouth or on the cast. In either case, a thin coat of resin must be carefully applied to the external surface of the housing and allowed to set in the pressure pot before the bulk of resin is added. This step is made necessary by the fine retentive groves and ridges on the ex-

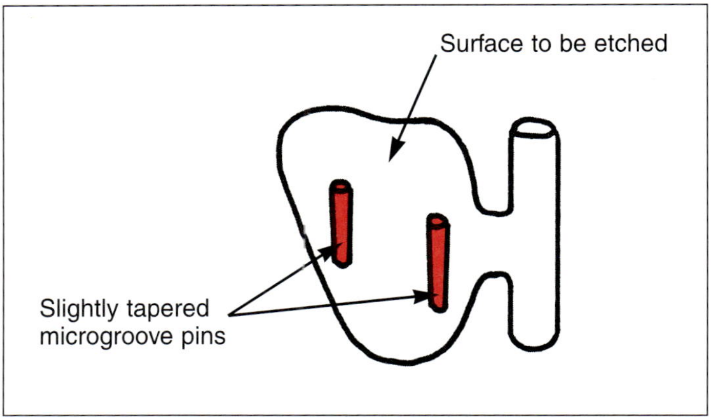

Fig 10-33 Internal view of resin-bonded pin attachment with microgrooves.

ternal of the housing. The quality of the joint between the housing and the partial is dependent on the highest-quality resin-metal interface. If a laboratory-grade repair resin (such as Perm by Caulk/Dentsply) is to be used, remember to remove the fibers. The fibers tend to clump when the resin is added using a brush. Once the resin has fully cured, additional, fibered resin is added to complete the attachment and the unit is placed back into the pressure pot. Later the bulk of the resin can be thinned appropriately to fit within the confines of the partial without damaging the interface. Autopolymerizing tooth-colored resin can also be used to reduce the risk of a show-through of the pink resin for those situations in which space is limited and esthetic demands are great. All internal traces of resin must be removed, preferably under magnification, after the processing unit is removed from the housing and before the retentive patrix is snapped into place.

The resilient attachment systems work best when their path of insertion/removal is restricted by the guiding planes prepared on the abutments and the well-fitting guide plates of the modern framework. When a restricted path of insertion exists, patients cannot jam the attachment to place from a variety of directions. They are limited to the path dictated by the planes. Patients must be advised that if they wish to minimize the wear and replacement of the resilient elements, they must place the attachment partial with their fingers only, never biting it to place. When the resilient component is forced to function only along its intended axis, the wear is greatly reduced, for both the ERA and the O-SO, as well as for any other modern attachment that uses a resilient insert. The manufacturers often show these attachments as being the only connection between the partial and the abutment teeth, implying that they function as an adequate rest system in addition to providing retention. It is my opinion that this approach breaks the basics of modern partial denture design and construction, and should therefore be ignored.

It has been implied that all extracoronal attachments are cast as a part of abutment crowns. This is not strictly true, as recent events have demonstrated the high level of success of resin-bonded extracoronal attachments (Fig 10-33). While it may not appear that an etched and bonded restoration would have sufficient retention to the tooth to resist the additional stress of an attachment, when microgroove preparation on the abutments is combined with careful patient selection, the bonded attachment is a successful and conservative means of obtaining the esthetics of an attachment system. A review of the work of Schärer and Marinello will acquaint the reader with the parameters of this therapy. In these cases especially, the partial denture should not load only the attachments. Additional abutments with positive rest preparations, either in natural tooth structure, crowns, or bonded surfaces, will reduce the load on the bonded attachment and should increase its length of service. All the extracoronal attachments discussed in this chapter are amenable to bonded restoration and have been used successfully over the last 8 to 10 years.

There are a variety of stud attachments that can be used for retention of the removable partial denture even though they are generally intended for the overdenture. The stud attachments, placed either in the endodontically prepared tooth or an implant, create potential problems for the precision attachment partial because their angulation is limited by the long axis of either base. They are to be placed first and the remainder of the guiding plane/attachment surfaces aligned with their long axis. If their alignment causes the other components to be directed beyond a usable limit, the use of the root or implant for retention should be rethought and these units used for occlusal stops only. A recent, and as yet not fully tested, system utilizing a ball that can swivel in a pressed fitting offers the promise of allowing a self-centering attachment to overcome alignment problems.

A mastery of these few attachment systems will cover the needs of most prosthodontists as well as provide a basis for the understanding of those systems to come. While the actual attachments can be expected to change and improve with time, the techniques for their use are standard and must be a part of the technical background of clinician and technician alike. The precision attachment, in combination with the other aspects of advanced partial denture construction, offers us the possibility of making prostheses that are esthetic, retentive, strong, and problem free, and that are undetectable by and will not compromise the oral health of the our patients.

Sources for Precision Attachments

Attachments International, Inc
600 S. Amphlett Blvd.
San Mateo, CA 94403
www.attachments.com/catalog

Cendres et Metaux SA
Rue de Boujean 122
Biel-Bienne 2501
Switzerland

Implant Innovations, Inc
4555 Riverside Drive
Palm Beach Gardens, FL 33410
www.3i-online.com

Preat Corporation
1120 Seventh Avenue
San Mateo, CA 94402
www.preat.com

Sterngold-ImplaMed
23 Frank Mossberg Drive
Box 839A
Attleboro, MA 02703
www.sterngold.com

11

Implants and Removable Partial Dentures

The advent of endosseous implants has dramatically changed our view of the complete denture, single tooth replacement, and full-mouth fixed restoration. Our successes in these areas have led to the consideration of obtaining implant support for the removable partial denture. The ideal use of one or more implants for the removable partial is to eliminate the distal extension base, especially in the mandible, where chronic problems associated with the loading of the edentulous ridge have plagued the profession. A second and more complex indication for their use is as a replacement for critical abutment teeth. An example is where a mandibular canine serving as a prime abutment is lost, leaving a lateral incisor as a terminal abutment. In the past, as described earlier, one might have considered a hinged major connector in this situation. A single implant placed in or near the canine position can provide both vertical support and, through the use of any of a number of attachment systems, retention as well. The future would appear bright for the use of selected implants, providing critical support for partial denture patients and still keeping the total cost of treatment at a reasonable level through the use of the removable partial denture as the prime restoration. The well-planned use of an isolated implant in these situations does not preclude a later, more complex treatment plan utilizing additional implants and fixed restorations.

Class I and II Situations

The obvious situation in which a single implant can make a major contribution to the success of a removable partial denture is in the distal extension partial denture. Patients have often been dissatisfied with our best efforts, either with conventional or precision attachment partials, because of chronic soreness under the distal extension base. This is especially true in those situations where the opposing arch contains a full complement of natural teeth or fixed partial dentures. When a complete denture is in-

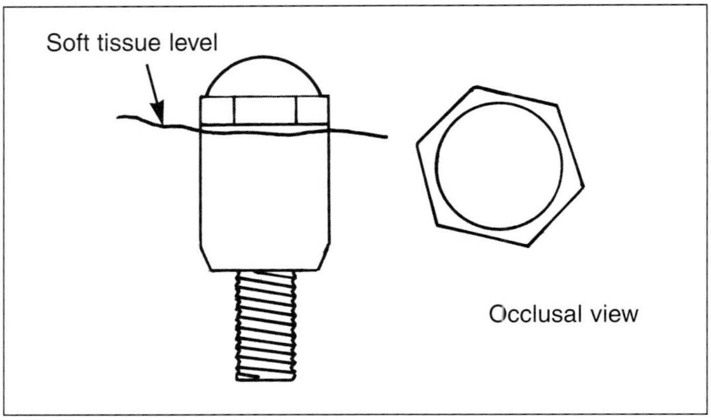

Fig 11-1 Lateral view of implant abutment without a center screw access (experimental).

volved, the potential load on the tissues is generally reduced and there are fewer patient complaints. Implants placed distal to the foramen, ideally in the area of the second molar, would effectively change the Class I or II situation to that of the Class III. The implant need not necessarily provide retention, since adequate retention is most always available from other abutments.

Unfortunately, because of long-term ridge resorption, finding sufficient bone in the distal extension base area becomes a major impediment to this therapy. Numerous studies have shown that implant loss is proportional to the length of the implants used, with special concern for the 7-mm implant, which is presently the shortest available. These studies have evaluated the implants for lateral support and retention as well as for vertical support. If the implants are used for vertical support only, the success of the shorter implants may well show better results. There are shorter implants that may be used in these situations. They are intended for extraoral maxillofacial use and are in the 3- to 4-mm range. They have not yet been evaluated for this purpose, but, again, when properly integrated and if not stressed laterally, they offer real potential. To cap the implant with a rounded abutment that would provide point contact on its most superior surface and no element of lateral contacts at all would allow vertical loading with minimal lateral stress. The partial denture connection to the abutment will need to be designed to provide the point contact and to maintain this contact throughout the life of the partial. A sliding point contact between the abutment and the partial would also allow the expansion and contraction of the mandible during opening and closing with minimum lateral forces being transmitted to the implant.

A problem arises with the use of any abutment that utilizes a center screw to engage the implant. The center point is the desired contact with the partial, and if that area bears the entire load, distortion of the centered screw head can be expected. With the use of a hexagonal configuration at the base of a rounded center contour, the unit can be torqued with a matching torque wrench, leaving the center of the ball stop for full contact (Fig 11-1). The hex is intended to lie at or just slightly above the soft tissue level.

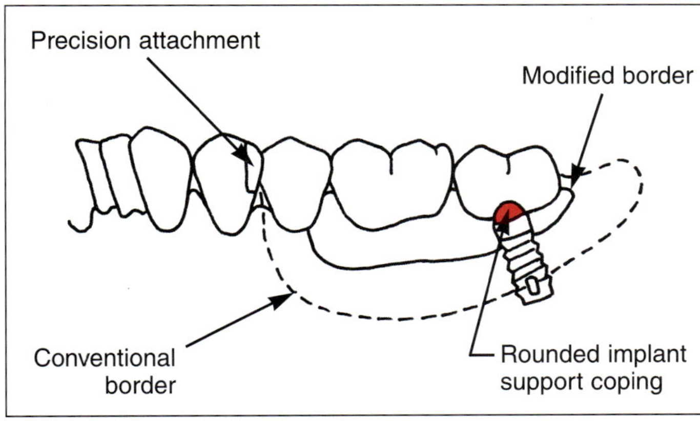

Fig 11-2 Modification of conventional denture borders with posterior implant support of Class I RPD.

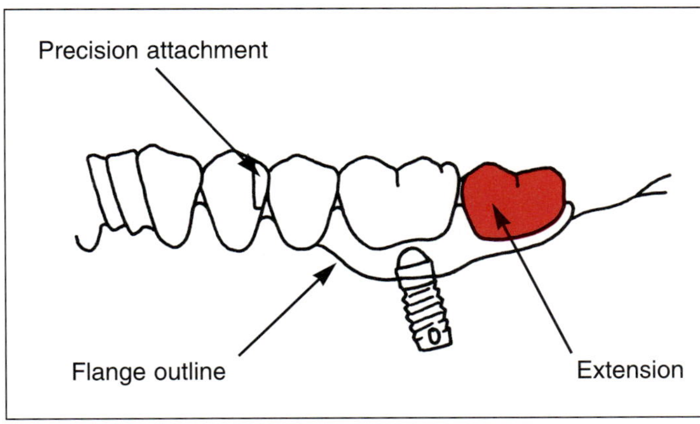

Fig 11-3 Posterior extension of one denture tooth beyond implant support.

It is quite possible that future advances in implant biomechanics will provide the profession with alternative forms of implants that will be subperiosteal rather than endosteal. Presently, a miniaturized subperiosteal implant, tentatively called an "on-plant," is being used experimentally in orthodontics and is under consideration for use with removable partial dentures. If the load on the implant can be made exclusively vertical, something of this type could be used in severely rebsorbed mandibles, eliminating or greatly reducing the need for grafting bone.

While the ideal position for Class I and II implant placement may be in the second molar area, any position distal to the terminal abutment where sufficient bone remains is acceptable. There is no reason for the denture base, when supported by an implant, to extend to the traditional borders. In fact, once posterior support is available, the design of the denture base should be altered to make its contours as much like those of a fixed restoration as possible (Fig 11-2). This will mean that there will be no advantage to extending into the floor of the mouth, or onto the external oblique ridge. It may well be possible to extend one occlusal unit posterior to the area of implant abutment support so that an implant placed in the second premolar position would support at least a first molar (Fig 11-3).

As long as the implant abutment is not expected to carry an attachment component, the angulation of the implant relative to the remaining abutments is not important. For those situations where some retentive attachment is required, the angulation is critical. The implant can be placed in the long axis of the remaining abutments (parallel to the path of insertion/removal), so that any attachment will draw with the remainder of the mouth, or the abutment, with its attachment component, must be completed first and the remainder of the mouth prepared to accept that path. The type of resilient attachments that would most often be used in this situation (ERA, O-SO, or similar) do allow for a small divergence from the path without damage to the resilient component. Recent additions to the available attachment systems, in particular the Sphero Flex (from the Rhein 83 Corp of Bologna, Italy, and available in North America from Preat Corp), offer swivel ball attachments that screw directly into the implant, allowing 8 degrees freedom of rotation. The retentive element is an O-ring much like that of the O-SO system.

Space may often be at a premium in those situations for which an attachment component is intended, especially if the implant is placed quite posteriorly. A measurement taken from the occlusal surface of the opposing tooth must show that space exists for the abutment, the attachment components, sufficient resin to pick up the attachment, and for the denture tooth destined to complete prosthesis. Where space is minimal, the occlusal surfaces of the denture tooth over the implant are protected with metal as in any attachment situation. If the implant is distal to the first molar, it is not essential that a denture tooth be placed where space is lacking. Occlusion through the first molar, when the base is well-supported posteriorly, will provide adequate mastication.

The implant-partial interface can be constructed in a number of ways. The possibility of using a modified healing abutment as the stop for the distal extension is certainly to be considered. A potential problem arises from the fact that the healing abutment is not to be torqued down to the same load as a transmucosal abutment would be. This means that screw loosening of the healing abutment can be expected and, indeed, that has been my experience. As long as the patient is aware of this possibility and inspects the healing abutment periodically, no damage is apt to occur should the abutment loosen. The modification of abutments that can receive greater torque should solve this problem for most situations, although at some increase in cost. A custom casting to the abutment or to the implant can be made to contain either an attachment component or the rounded occlusal stop. These can be made using the hexed UCLA-type castable abutment or by modifying any of the ball abutments normally used for overdentures. Contour modifications of these attachments would be done on the working cast so that the angulation of the sides of the rounded occlusal stops would be in general alignment with the guiding planes planned for other abutments. This step will reduce the need for excessive blockout on the partial.

The clinician must choose between making a custom metal casting to ride on the ball (rounded occlusal stop) or to allow that contact to be in the resin of the denture base. For the former, implant analogues will have to be present on the master cast for the partial denture casting. They may be needed on the working cast for any fixed

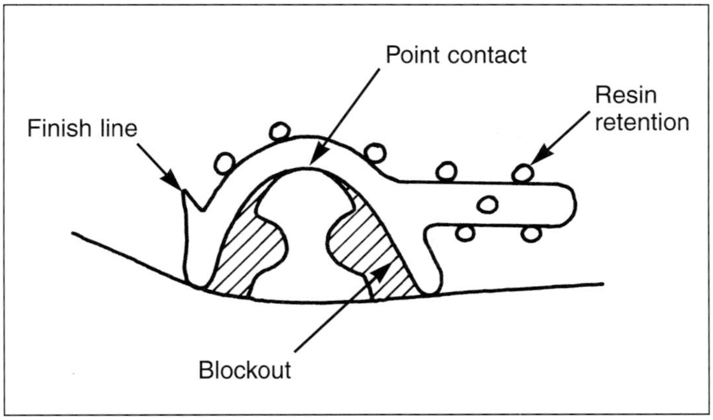

Fig 11-4 Design of overcoping for implant stud attachment.

components as well. On the master cast, the patrix (ie, the ball) is blocked out so that only the center of the ball surface will be contacted; this unit is duplicated in refractory (Fig 11-4). An overcasting is waxed with retentive beads or loops to lock the casting into the denture base if the overcasting is to be retained with resin alone. A tang extension, running to the retentive meshwork, will also be required so that the casting can be picked up from the mouth after the framework is fitted. In situations where space is limited, the tang extensions can be soldered to the retentive meshwork of the partial denture casting.

The anterior retentive components of implant-supported distal extension partial dentures need not offer any stress relief as they should with the conventional Class I and II situations. Either intracoronal or extracoronal attachments or conventional clasping can be used effectively, since these partials are now all "tooth"-supported.

The other major area of interest is that in which the implant becomes a prime retentive abutment, as it would if a canine were to be replaced by an implant. In these situations, we are going to be faced with decisions on the best way to integrate the implant into the support, stability, and retention of the partial denture. We will also need to consider the esthetic replacement of the missing tooth that would be found over the implant in question.

Perhaps the easiest approach will always be to place an attachment on the implant, either connecting directly to the implant or threaded onto the transmucosal abutment. Given sufficient space, any stud-type attachment could be used along with the ERA– and O-SO–type systems. The attachment need only fit within the shape of the replacement tooth and allow metal retentive extensions from the framework that will provide dependable retention for the denture tooth and associated denture base resin. When space is very limited, as one might find in a severe Class II Div II case, it may be necessary to place a single tooth on the implant and use that unit as a conventional or attachment abutment. We have little experience in this area as yet, and cannot predict the prognosis of tying this implant abutment to the partial through the implant crown.

When using the implant crown as a conventional abutment tooth, the partial framework must be intimately in contact with all remaining abutment teeth, natural or crowned, so that the teeth will be effectively splinted to the implant. The fact that the implant crown will not change its position in the arch while the remaining natural teeth have the potential to migrate should not complicate the design if the partial fits to our standards and is worn by the patient on a daily basis. Should the partial not be worn for any lengthy period, this disparity in the possible migration of the abutments could result in a framework that no longer fully seats.

For these single implant abutment crowns, the use of an extracoronal attachment to retain the partial denture seems indicated. Intracoronal attachments will most likely not be possible because the internal contour of the crown is taken up by the implant components. The selection of the attachment to be added to the implant crown is driven by both the design of the implant and the needs of the partial denture. Since the implant crown, properly integrated, will not move, there will be some need to consider stress relief if the partial in question is a Class I. The potential lever arm is an issue here as it would be for any cantilever from a terminal implant. Unfortunately, there is no specific body of knowledge to which to refer at this time to help us with our decisions on stress relief. We will have to draw on our experience with other implant prostheses as well as conventional knowledge of the removable partial denture. For Class I situations, in the mandible at least, it would appear that if there is no possibility of posterior implant support, then the more resilient the attachment, the less the possible damage to the implant. This would suggest a ball attachment with an O-ring retentive element placed extracoronally as the best possible option. Obviously, conventional clasping with resilient wire forms will also offer stress relief depending on the amount of relief built into the casting.

Class III and IV Situations

We would expect implants in Class III and IV situations to be used as overdenture abutments, usually with some type of attachment system for retention of the partial. When two or more implants can be splinted together with a bar, a clip-retained partial offers a dependable option. The bar-clip assembly can be used with any other attachment system, conventional clasping on other teeth, and with precision milled crowns to provide both lateral stability and retention. Since the parallelism of multiple implants cannot be assured, the bar-clip system allows any undercuts in the gold cylinders to be blocked out in the housing and not be contacted by the partial casting (Fig 11-5). The superior surface of the bar can always be used as a vertical stop for the partial so that the implant attachments need take no wear at all from the housing.

The lack of vertical space for the implant attachment system will always be a potential source of problems. For that reason alone, a diagnostic waxing and set-up is essential. This procedure must contain an evaluation of the implant attachment mechanism, best accomplished by placing the implant components on the diagnostic cast after a putty matrix has been made from the diagnostic set-up so that the ac-

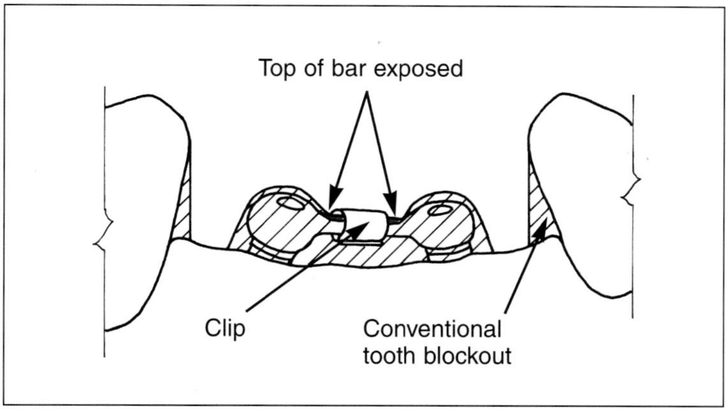

Fig 11-5 Blockout of implant bar-clip for cast partial denture framework.

tual remaining space can be clearly identified. This step will also allow the clinician to decide if metal occlusal surfaces on the denture teeth will be required to protect the attachment system, since the addition of these surfaces will be a factor in the final cost of treatment.

While the use of implants in conjunction with removable partial dentures is in its infancy, the chances are excellent that new systems and new uses for those systems will enter our practices in the future. As long as implants are used in conjunction with thorough mouth preparation of soft and hard tissues, employ precisely fitting castings, and are cared for with regular recall and appropriate maintenance, we can be confident that they will improve the quality of removable prosthodontic therapy. To expect them to be a solution for all our problems without this level of careful adherence to basic principles is foolhardy.

Index

D

E

F